Arthritis:
Secrets of Natural Healing

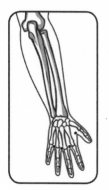 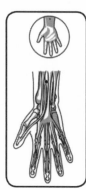 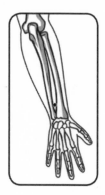

Arthritis:
Secrets of Natural Healing

Mao Shing Ni, Ph.D., D.O.M., L.Ac.

and

Jason Moskovitz, M.A.T.C.M., Dipl.O.M., L.Ac.

TAO OF
WELLNESS
PRESS
Los Angeles

Published by
Tao of Wellness Press
An Imprint of SevenStar Communications
13315 W. Washington Boulevard, Suite 200
Los Angeles, CA 90066
www.taoofwellness.com

Ni, Mao Shing.

      Arthritis : secrets of natural healing / by Mao Shing Ni and Jason Moskovitz. -- Los Angeles : Tao of Wellness Press, c2012.

             p. ; cm.

             ISBN: 978-1-887575-34-8
             Includes index.

             1. Arthritis--Alternative treatment. 2. Arthritis--Diet therapy. 3. Medicine, Chinese. 4. Herbs--Therapeutic use. I. Moskovitz, Jason. II. Title. III. Title: Arthritis.

RC933 .N5 2012

616.7/2206--dc23   1203

Cover design and photographs by Justina Krakowski
Figure drawings by Peter Zaslav
Editing, page layout and design by Meagan Brusnighan

A note to readers:
This book is intended to be informational and should not be considered a substitute for advice from a medical professional, whom the reader should consult before beginning any diet or exercise regiment, and before taking any dietary supplements or other medications. The author and publisher expressly disclaim responsibility for any adverse effects arising from the use or application of the information contained in this book.

Table of Contents

Chapter Two: | 37
Diet and Nutrition

Chapter Four: | 121
Joint Care, Exercise, and Acupressure

Chapter Five: | 177
Your Mind, Stress and Inflammation

Introduction

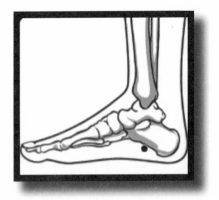

The Wakeup Call

Pain is universal. It's your body's way of letting you know that something is wrong. This signal usually begins with inflammation. Acute inflammation is a normal process that protects and heals the body following physical injury or infection. But if the source causing the inflammation continues for an extended period of time, the inflammation becomes chronic. Chronic inflammation can result from a viral or bacterial infection, an autoimmune reaction, environmental factors like pollen or dust, or a constant trigger of inflammatory molecules.

In the case of arthritis, pain is typically noticeable after the joint has already started to wear down and begun to cause chronic inflammation. Joint capsules have little nerve supply to them, but directly outside of the capsules are bones, which have an abundant supply of nerves. This is where your brain receives pain signals from when something inside the capsule becomes damaged, such as faulty or torn cartilage.

When your body communicates pain, it's giving you an opportunity to learn something about yourself. Maybe you need to move differently? Maybe your diet of refined starch and sugar is causing a health breakdown? Maybe you are stuck emotionally with unhappiness, anger or despair? Often, our lives are so busy that a nagging pain will only motivate us to make it disappear as quickly as possible. Taking the usual painkillers may work for the moment, but what happened to the lesson?

It's like driving down the freeway when your car's engine warning light comes on, but instead of pulling over to examine the engine, you take out a hammer to knock out the warning light and continue driving. Let's be honest, it's probably unthinkable for most of us to ignore a warning light in our car. But how often have we done that with our bodies, simply ignoring signs of impending sickness or the warning for us to slow down? Probably too often to count!

Pain is invisible. Pain doesn't show up on an X-ray or imaging scan. The moment a new arthritic pain is felt there is likely not going to be any imaging that shows something is physically wrong unless there's an obvious tear or break. But over time, most pains can develop into inflammation or degeneration that's visible on an X-ray or MRI.

Nature's Amazing Design

The human body is a truly awesome creation. Like an ecosystem unto itself, the many cells and processes that make up your body work synergistically for its survival and longevity. Your blood vessels act like an irrigation system. They move blood, oxygen, and other chemicals to the farthest reaches of your body. Your nervous system works like an electrical grid, carrying information in every direction so you can respond appropriately. And your joints are the intersections these messages and materials must pass through to reach their destination. The joints also allow you to walk, run, jump, squat, grab, and climb.

You use your joints for your job, for your family, and for having fun. Some of these uses bring productivity and joy. Other uses are simply a by-product of your responsibilities: carrying groceries, lifting children, sitting in meetings, climbing stairs, harvesting crops, and building shelter. When your joints are used, your body responds in the best way it knows to maintain their health, by pumping body fluids into the joints to keep them refreshed. Your breathing and heart rates are regulated to supply your joints with their unique energy requirements. So how did your joints end up in this state? Life throws many monkey wrenches at the joints. Repetitive movements, incorrect postures, accidents or even lack of movement can lead to symptoms like joint pain and stiffness that is generally labeled as arthritis. But there are, in fact, more than 100 types of arthritis. Many other factors affect joint health as well, including diet, exercise, weight, trauma, infectious disease, environment and genetics.

Unfortunately, many people falsely think arthritis pain is a normal part of life. People are quick to lump arthritis together with illnesses like heart disease and cancer, expecting any of these to pop up at some point in life because, as many say, "I'm getting older." This couldn't be further from reality. We have witnessed many of our patients in their 70s, 80s, and even 90s playing tennis, golfing and jogging regularly without arthritic pain. Yes, your body has limits and you must exercise care and caution in how you use it, but expecting disease merely because you are getting older is pointless.

Arthritis can affect many different people and at any age. Young children develop juvenile arthritis due to bacterial or viral infections, women around menopause may suffer from arthritis and osteoporosis, and older people may come down with arthritic pain or mobility issues due, not necessarily to their age, but as a result of a lifetime of poor habits, diseases, or diminished health. To accept arthritic pain as you age is to prepare yourself for more suffering, a less active lifestyle and even depression.

Integrative Solutions for Arthritis Sufferers

New solutions are available for the millions of arthritis sufferers who have exhausted the typical treatments. There are always new drugs on the market, and surgical procedures are being constantly improved and refined. However, these seemingly advanced technologies have yet to stand the test of time, and are usually associated with side effects. The solutions that we advocate, however, are actually quite old. Traditional Chinese medicine – with its wide range of therapies including acupuncture, bodywork, herbal and nutritional therapies, and exercise regimens – has been treating arthritis and refining its approach to the disease for thousands of years. In the Chinese medical classics there are countless cases of crippled arthritic patients successfully overcoming their condition. These patients used Chinese medicine and enjoyed an active lifestyle while practicing Tai Chi, playing sports, and making preventative daily choices about food and lifestyle that keep their minds and bodies vibrant and pain-free for much of their lives.

We have certainly seen the recovery first hand in our patients and we know that you can too. If you are interested in healing your arthritis naturally, we have a comprehensive program for you in this book. In the following chapters you will discover how to identify the different types of arthritis and how to care for it through diet and nutrition, herbal therapy, bodywork, acupressure, and exercise therapy. You will learn about the mind-body connection and how stress affects the pain and inflammation in your body, as well as the natural ways to reduce your tension and therefore, your inflammation. We also explore the environmental factors that can contribute to your pain. Finally, we guide you in how to assemble your healing team by identifying the right open-minded healthcare professionals who are willing to collaborate with others to serve your needs. Imagine a team comprising of a nutritionist, physical therapist, exercise trainer, internist, rheumatologist, acupuncturist, and Chinese medical doctors all working together to ensure your proper healing and wellbeing. This is the Tao of Wellness way.

If this sounds good to you, we invite you to read on.

Using this Book

Educating and empowering yourself during times of pain or disease can feel challenging. But investing in the healing process described in this book is crucial for a faster and more complete recovery. You'll discover many resources here to help you eliminate arthritic pain and revive your lifestyle.

The way Chinese medicine treats arthritis will be covered, and so will the way arthritis is defined and treated in Western medicine. This way you can work more easily with your Eastern and Western doctors in constructing the best plan for you. While there is enough self-care information provided here to carry you out of arthritic disorders, success is best achieved when your doctor of acupuncture and Chinese medicine guides you through a customized process.

Studies show that regular acupuncture treatments can reduce the symptoms of arthritis and assist the body's own natural regenerative power. This is most important in healing the articular cartilage at the ends of bones. The more chronic and degenerative the state of arthritis, the more difficult this healing can be. For the best results, get treatments early and consistently. Relief is available to anyone who is proactive and participates in their own healing process along with guidance from a competent healing team.

Chapter One:
The Many Faces of
Arthritis

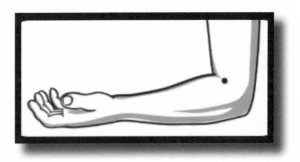

Your entrance into joint pain may have happened in an instant, or it may have been building for some time, developing gradually like a dim light slowly turning itself on. It's possible you've had pain since you were a child, but there are also many who don't experience arthritis until later in life. Regardless of your circumstance, discovering what kind of pain or immobility you have will certainly help in guiding your care.

The phenomenon of arthritis is as old as human history. The wear and tear on the body, particularly the joints, resulted from hunting, farming, and labor-intensive activities which left our ancestors in debilitating pain. This prompted a search for relief and understanding about how arthritis progresses. In conventional medicine, the paradigm that arthritis is due to inflammation has led to the use of anti-inflammatory drugs and surgery as the predominant methods of treatment. However, as any sufferer of arthritis will readily acknowledge, these treatments are often temporary, far from completely satisfactory, and are often loaded with side effects.

Over the course of its five thousand years of continuous use, Chinese medicine has recognized that there are other factors at work besides injuries and wear and tear. These factors include invasive pathogens, environmental factors and depletion of essence or inadequate nutrition. Modern research has only just begun to validate and appreciate the wisdom of the East; such as the discovery that bacterial, viral, fungal and parasitic infections may be the cause of many cases of arthritis, that environmental toxins and changing weather patterns may contribute to inflammation, and that deficiency in nutrients like vitamin D can also lead to erosion of bones and joints.

Genetic Predisposition and Epigenetics

Genetics play a role in, but aren't considered to be a factor for more than 30% of arthritis sufferers. Usually there is someone in the family who has arthritis, whether it is osteoarthritis, gout, or rheumatoid arthritis. However, even if that applies to you, don't feel that you are doomed to develop it. A branch of genetic science called epigenetics has shown that all genes require a trigger for it to express. That means that if you have a genetic predisposition to develop arthritis, you have the power to prevent its expression. For example, you can choose to eat a diet rich in omega fatty acids that lower inflammation in your body. In essence, genetics can be a component in developing arthritis, but it doesn't have to happen to you.

The Unaffordable Toll of Arthritis

Arthritis is the number one cause of disability in the United States. The Centers for Disease Control report that 46 million Americans have been diagnosed with arthritis. Some sources put the number higher, claiming that closer to 60 million Americans suffer from some type of arthritis. Half of all arthritis sufferers are over 65 years old, and women past the age of 45 are more likely than men their age to develop arthritis. By 2030 it's estimated that arthritis sufferers will increase 46% to represent 67 million Americans. Annually, arthritis is responsible for 44 million doctor's visits and nearly one million hospitalizations. In 2003, arthritis cost the U.S. $128 billion. That accounts for $81 billion in medical costs and $47 billion in lost wages. This represented 1.2% of the U.S. gross domestic product for 2003. 1.2% of anything may not seem like much, but for a nation as large as the U.S., arthritis is a widespread problem that carries a substantial price tag, not to mention the physical and emotional toll that the disease places on the individual sufferer.

Fortunately for those living with arthritis, more integrative wellness programs involving Chinese medicine, lifestyle and nutritional modification are becoming available to patients every year, leading to improved quality of life, increased productivity and reduced medical cost.

Let's take a look at the different faces of arthritis in the following pages. Perhaps you can relate to one or more of these.

Anatomy of a Joint – Getting a Lay of the Land

What's inside a joint? The joint capsule is a membrane that surrounds the outside of the joint, connecting adjacent bones to one another. It contains many nerve endings but has no blood or lymph vessels. The lack of these vessels makes joint nourishment and repair much slower than in other parts of the body.

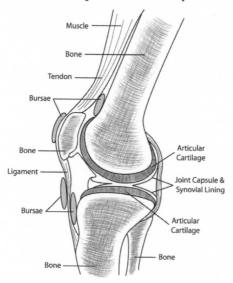

The synovial lining is the inside layer of the joint capsule. It secretes synovial fluid that lubricates the joint and sends in nutrients.

Ligaments are bands of strong tissue that connect bones to one another, positioned to stabilize their movement. You'll often hear of someone tearing their ACL. That's the anterior cruciate ligament and is a common site of soft tissue injury in the knee.

Tendons are tough fibrous tissues connecting muscles to bones, allowing the muscle to control the bone's movement while also stabilizing the joint.

Muscles are tissues that contract and expand so we can use our bones and joints. Muscles also serve as supplemental shock absorption.

Bursae are fluid-filled sacs positioned around the joint to protect tendons and ligaments from the friction of their use. Without them, tendons and ligaments would rub against the adjacent bone, wearing them away.

Articular cartilage is the tough rubbery connective tissue that covers the ends of bones at their point of friction. Imbalance or injury in any part of the joint can cause discomfort. Pain may quickly scare someone into thinking their cartilage has worn away. While this is possible, you'll want a thorough examination to determine exactly from where your source of pain is coming.

The Cushions of Your Bones: the Wear and Tear of Cartilage

Cartilage serves as the joint's primary shock absorber. It's made mostly of water and is very slippery, allowing bones to slide easily across one other. Pain due to osteoarthritis occurs primarily because this cartilage wears away. But pain is not always the first sign to show up. Stiffness or lack of mobility can also be a warning sign that the cartilage is starting to break down. Cartilage doesn't have a ready supply of blood or nerves, which means that its growth and repair takes much longer than other tissues. When injured, cartilage will often regenerate itself slowly and in poorer quality, and may even be replaced by stiff scar tissue. Certain cartilage cells responsible for its repair will produce chemicals that breakdown the faulty cartilage. Often, completely normal cartilage will also be removed by these chemicals if this mechanism isn't appropriately shut down.

Proper self-care in conjunction with the body's natural healing processes should keep the cartilage from losing its quality, even later in life. It's when the destructive processes overtake your efforts to maintain healthy joints that things take a turn for the worse. Conventional medicine has yet to find an effective way to accomplish the balance required by this cartilage life cycle. Cartilage loss is a problem that can't be solved with the mediation of one chemical process, as is the attempt of most modern drugs. One pill will likely never be enough to solve the issue. This natural immune response, which includes many simultaneous processes, requires an equally diverse system of support. Chinese medicine is one of the only medical systems whose whole-person approach can match the unique presentation of a person's arthritis. Of course, the cornerstone of healing arthritis should always start with exercise, nutrition, and lifestyle change.

Joint Injury – the Beginning of Arthritis

Trauma is a common cause of osteoarthritis, usually from repeated injury. A career as a football player can be quite damaging to the upper spine, thanks to the thousands of hard impacts a player takes to the head and neck. A field worker who bends over at the waist for long hours can develop arthritis of the lower spinal vertebrae. Inventions such as the car, computer, and chair have millions of people assuming a similar seated posture for hours at a time every day. These types of activities put varying degrees of stress on the joints, but self-care should be equally important, no matter what kind of job or activity is wearing down your joints. However, what works best for one person might hold much less value with someone else. Getting an individualized treatment plan from your acupuncturist is always advised before embarking on a healing regimen. Occupational and physical therapists can evaluate how you live and work. If recreational activities like tennis or soccer are the culprit, then make sure to work with an experienced coach or instructor to prevent accidents or a re-injury.

Osteoarthritis, the Most Common Arthritis

Osteoarthritis (OA) is the most common form of arthritis. It primarily affects weight bearing joints, such as the hips and knees. It can also cause problems in the hands, feet, and spine. OA is a result of either misuse or overuse of a joint. Osteoarthritis is considered to be a disease, but it's more appropriate to think of it as an injury. OA leads to large, stiff, painful joints, and will often affect one side of the body more severely than the other.

When cartilage at the end of bones becomes thin, it creates a bone-on-bone joint, and the makings of osteoarthritis. Other disorders may develop at the same time, such as bone spurs, which can invade the joint space and create intense pain. However it happens, once the cartilage is gone, the underlying bone may start to degrade as well. This will cause the immune system to rebuild more bone in place of the worn out cartilage. But when this happens, even walking or standing can become painful enough to discourage movement. Less movement will lead to atrophy of the surrounding tissues, creating a downward spiral of pain, weakness and disability.

Diagnosis of OA is primarily arrived at by examining the patient's history, performing a physical exam, and taking an x-ray, though the correlation is not always accurate. Around 40% of patients with the worst x-ray classification for osteoarthritis are pain-free.

The root of osteoarthritis is the destruction of chondrocytes, the cells that make cartilage. The logical way to solve this problem lies in building up substances in the joint that are chondro-protective and chondro-regenerative, and by simultaneously reducing inflammation in the degenerative joint. Such substances provide arthritis pain management and relief for joint pain and inflammation without harming the joint itself. These days, people are finding help in acupuncture, Chinese medicine and nutrition, and Tai Chi.

Gout, the Rich Person's Disease

Historically, gout was a "rich person's" disease because it took excess meat and alcohol (foods that, traditionally, only the rich could afford) to produce the characteristic gout pain. This pain usually settles in the large joint of the big toe and is a result of hyperuricemia, otherwise known as excess uric acid in the blood. Uric acid crystals, waste products from protein metabolism, deposit themselves in the joint and surrounding tissues of the big toe, or other joints of the body. This is commonly due to lifestyle factors including obesity, a lack of exercise, and a diet rich in alcohol, sugar, and meat. The joint will become swollen, red, and very painful. Other possible triggers for gout include insulin resistance and high blood pressure, so consult your physician to determine your cause. Oxalic acid in the body can also be confused with gout. However, oxalic acid comes from eating excessive amounts of spinach, chard, or chocolate, and can deposit in the kidneys as stones or end up, like gout, in the joints. Chinese medical treatment calls for diet change, herbal and nutritional therapies, acupuncture, and lifestyle modification as a solution. Drinking 8-10 glasses of water per day is recommended, both for prevention and during episodes of gout attack.

Ankylosing Spondylitis—Arthritis of the Spine

There are many possible causes of back pain, and one of them is arthritis of the spine. This condition is called ankylosing spondylitis (AS), which means an arthritic inflammation of the spine that may result in fusion of the vertebrae. The arthritis may cause growth in the vertebrae that ends up fusing two or more vertebrae together, which leads to pain, stiffness, and difficulty moving. AS also often involves the sacroiliac joint, which is the joint between the spine and the pelvis. Inflammation and stiffness in this joint can make even daily movements like walking, turning in bed, bending over to pick up an object, or even tie your shoe incredibly painful.

The cause for AS is unknown but it is often observed that AS is triggered by intestinal infections. These patients often suffer from chronic digestive symptoms that may include abdominal pain, diarrhea, constipation, bloating and excess flatulence. Medical conditions like inflammatory bowel diseases and celiac disorders must be treated promptly. Genetics also seem to play a role in AS. About 40% of AS sufferers test positive for a genetic marker in their blood called HLA-B27. You might discover a family history of this; perhaps an uncle, grandparent or cousin also suffered from AS.

Conventional treatment for Ankylosing spondylitis involves medication, exercise, and physical therapy. In severe cases surgery may be recommended, but it's considered to be risky. Acupuncture, electrical stimulation, far-infrared heat therapy, along with nutrition and herbal therapies, have also been effectively used for managing the symptoms and condition of AS, and are safer than surgery.

Why We Get Shorter (and Other Pains of Discs, Spurs, and Stenosis)

The human spine is made up of 33 bones called vertebrae, which are separated by discs made from a gelatinous material to cushion and lessen pressure in your spine. This gelatinous material, known as cartilage, functions like gel pads in your shoes. With normal wear and tear, as well as injuries to the spine from auto accidents, sports traumas, and falls and improper posture, the discs may suffer tears, splits, or protrusions, leading to compression of your nerves. Scar tissue from your body's repair process can also impinge on the nerve endings, as can bony growths called bone spurs. Moreover, the narrowing of the spinal canal, or spinal stenosis due to disc degeneration, can further complicate this problem. This condition is generally called degenerative disc disease (DDD) and results in pain, stiffness, and numbness in the neck, back, hips, and legs and can drastically reduce the sufferer's quality of life. To add insult to injury, since discs help maintain space between the vertebrae, when discs degenerate and flatten, it contributes to a decrease in height. It's no wonder that as we get older, we also get shorter. Conventional treatments may include surgery, epidural injections, medication and physical therapy. Acupuncture, herbal and nutritional therapies, along with gentle exercises like Tai Chi and Qi Gong, can often help reduce pain and inflammation, strengthen the back and the abdomen, and increase range of motion.

Rheumatoid Arthritis

Rheumatoid arthritis (RA), along with lupus and psoriatic arthritis, is one of the most prevalent forms of autoimmune disorders to present with joint pain. An autoimmune disorder results when the body's immune system malfunctions and attacks itself, like mutinous soldiers on the battlefield firing on their former command. Rheumatoid arthritis tends to affect the body symmetrically, meaning both hands or both knees will look and feel similar. Rheumatic joints are typically red, swollen, warm, and spongy to the touch. Unlike osteoarthritis, RA symptoms can come and go frequently and can often be accompanied by symptoms like fatigue, fever, anemia, and feelings of sickness in addition to related disorders of the skin, lungs, kidneys, liver, eyes, bones, nerves, and blood vessels.

Western medicine employs non-steroidal anti-inflammatory drugs (NSAIDs), corticosteroids, and methotrexate, which are of some benefit but are extremely toxic and can result in further damage to the bones and joints. Aspirin is an old favorite that's prescribed on a daily basis by most physicians. But while aspirin has proven effective in reducing the pain of RA, long-term use can negatively impact the gastrointestinal tract and blood vessels. Possible symptoms include nausea, indigestion, loss of appetite, ulcers, and hemorrhage. But even a broken immune system can do some of its other jobs, such as repelling bacteria, viruses, and other pathogens, all of which have a much easier time entering the body when the immune system is shut down with drugs.

Any physician's primary goal should be to treat the patient in the least harmful way. Fortunately, thanks to a mountain of evidence, we know that a specific combination of systemic herbal nutrients, acupuncture, enzymes, and nutritional supplementation may be the best medicines for difficult to treat inflammatory joint conditions. An acupuncturist will often diagnose RA as a combination of arthritis subtypes according to Chinese medicine. Each of these subtypes comes with a specific and effective treatment protocol.

Lupus Arthritis

Lupus is short for Systemic Lupus Erythematosus (SLE), which is a type of autoimmune condition. Lupus can affect the joints as well as the skin and organs. Most sufferers develop some joint pain, often in the fingers, hands, wrists, and knees. The most visible symptom, which affects half of Lupus sufferers, is a red rash over the nose and cheeks that looks like a butterfly covering the face. Other common symptoms include fatigue and fever. But other organs can be affected, including the heart, kidneys, and lungs. Most patients receive no explanation of how Lupus and most other autoimmune conditions are caused, but it is often observed that a stressful lifestyle can deplete the body to a point where the immune system is not only weakened but starts behaving erratically and attacks itself. Conventional medicine doesn't yet have effective solutions for Lupus other than steroids and immunosuppressant drugs. Chinese medicine has recognized that many Lupus conditions originate with an invasive pathogen that causes disarray in the immune system, and therefore seeks to rebalance the immune system by eliminating pathogenic toxins and reducing inflammation. Long-term relief must come from a comprehensive approach like those outlined in this book.

Psoriatic Arthritis

Psoriasis is a chronic autoimmune condition that affects the skin, most commonly appearing as scaly white patches on the skin of the elbows and knees caused by an overgrowth of skin cells, but any part of the body can be affected. This "faulty" condition, seen in 2-3% of the global population, is caused by an immune system that is sending out the wrong signals and, in effect, attacking otherwise healthy parts of the body, including joints. In this case, it's not wear and tear that brings on the arthritis but an internal inflammatory response to the excessive immune activity. For every 10 people with psoriasis, one to three develop psoriatic arthritis simultaneously. Many triggers can bring on psoriasis, including stress, allergies, diet, climate, medications, and even injury to the skin. Since the problem originates with the immune system, effective treatments must target the hyperactive immune system through an elimination of triggers while also modulating its function. Our clinical experience has shown that diet in particular plays a large role in the eventual remission of the disease. When we put patients on a plant-based diet free of any animal products, coupled with weekly acupuncture and herbal therapy, a majority of our patients experienced dramatic relief within three months.

Heart Disease and Arthritis

Arthritis and heart disease often occur simultaneously. In fact, a recent study found that arthritis affects 57 percent of adults with heart disease. For people with rheumatoid arthritis, RA is now known to be a separate risk factor for heart disease, similar to cholesterol. All people with arthritis should be aware of their increased risk for heart disease. The risk of cardiovascular disease (CVD) for people with RA has been found to be comparable to the risk of CVD in people with type 2 diabetes. It is important for people with RA, as well as other inflammatory disorders, such as ankylosing spondylitis, lupus, and reactive arthritis, to make dietary and lifestyle changes to reduce cardiovascular risk factors. Modifying such risk factors – that is, quitting smoking and lowering cholesterol and blood pressure – could help reduce the increased risk of cardiovascular problems in people with RA.

Allergies and Arthritis

A sensitive immune system can be sparked into action at the change of season or simply by pollen or common foods. The inflammation seen in red, itchy eyes during an allergy attack can also cause joint pain to worsen. Mucus can flow and thicken as a way to clean out allergens, but those same fluids can accumulate internally in the joints and add to soreness. The joints need a swift-moving fluid environment to keep them healthy. Repetitive allergic reactions can get fluids and inflammation on overdrive to the point that joints can develop pain or inflammation as a result. That's the reason why some arthritis sufferers experience flare-ups during hay fever season when their allergies act up.

Allergy tests should be performed to discover which allergens may be causing a reaction. Avoidance of the offending foods or environments can usually reduce the allergic reaction. If that's not possible or fails to arrest the allergy, conventional treatments may include weekly allergy shots taken over a period of time. Additionally, over-the-counter drugs such as antihistamines, decongestants, and pain-relievers may be recommended for symptomatic relief.

However, many people find allergy shots tedious and antihistamines' effect temporary at best. Increasing numbers of people are finding longer lasting relief from acupuncture, nutrition and herbal therapies. Acupuncture can be used to "reprogram" the immune system by modulating its response to allergens. Treatment with an experienced practitioner can help improve your immune system's ability to confront and clear away allergens and inflammation. That way, what could have been an indefinite avoidance of a favorite food or climate can eventually be reversed and appreciated once again. And the best part is the arthritis won't flare up.

Don't Let it Tick You Off – Lyme Disease and Arthritis

More and more people are coming into our offices with rashes, acute swelling and inflammation of their joints coupled with fatigue, headache, and other debilitating symptoms. Upon inquiry, we find a history of tick bites or travels to tick-infested areas, such as the Northeast, around the Great Lakes, or Northern California. A blood test for Lyme disease usually comes back positive for infection. Lyme disease is caused by a bacterium called Borrelia carried by certain ticks. When these infected ticks bite and feed on their human host, they can transmit the bacteria within 1-2 days. Conventional treatment is a specific course of antibiotics. If that fails, patients are left managing their illness with anti-inflammatory and pain-relieving drugs. The bacterium responsible for Lyme infection and the resulting arthritis is not always responsive to antibiotics, and as with most other bacteria, it can build a resistance to the antibiotics and render the drugs ineffective. At the Tao of Wellness our approach to Lyme disease is to support the immune system so that your natural defenses can be developed to combat the bacteria and reduce the inflammatory process. The treatment program consists of acupuncture, tuina bodywork, cupping to stimulate the lymphatic system, and far-infrared heat treatments to increase circulation in the joint spaces and help eliminate toxins. Diet, nutrition, and herbal therapies help to support your body to function optimally and aid in the recovery with the use of essential foods, nutrients, and natural bacteria-inhibiting and vitality-boosting herbs.

Chronic Fatigue Syndrome and Arthritis

There are conditions that frustrate conventional medicine and have puzzled clinicians for decades without ever reaching a consensus about what these conditions are or how to treat them. Chronic fatigue syndrome, which affects an estimated 4 million people in the United States alone, is one of these baffling conditions. It causes a long-standing general weakness accompanied by fatigue, decreased concentration, memory loss, poor digestion, sleep disorders, depression, frequent colds, yeast infections, and joint and muscle pain.

Recent studies show that certain viral infections, like Epstein-Barr Virus (EBV), Cytomegalo Virus (CMV), or Parvovirus can bring on chronic fatigue; so can overexertion and long-standing illnesses. But infection can also challenge and weaken the immune system enough to leave a lasting fatigue that's otherwise unexplainable. A chronic infection that leads to an immune system breakdown can result in weak, flaccid muscles, tendons, ligaments, and joints.

However, a full recovery from chronic fatigue syndrome is possible with a treatment of acupuncture and Chinese medicine. Our approach is to focus on the basics: plenty of rest and sleep, good nutrition, a gradual build-up of exercise, and a low stress lifestyle to support healthy immune function. Remember not to overdo your exercise routine. We start most patients with 15 minutes of gentle exercise, such as brisk walking, each day for a week before increasing the exercise by five additional minutes each week, depending on how the patient feels. Within two to three months, most patients are exercising for 45 minutes daily.

A majority of illnesses that get the "chronic" label can take time to show noticeable improvement. Be patient, stick to the treatment course set out by your practitioner, and most definitely minimize overexertion and get immediate treatment when you get sick.

Rebecca's Story

Rebecca's pain began one morning as she was getting out of bed. She said it felt as if the inside of her joints were on fire. It went away quickly, so she assumed it was just lingering soreness from her daily workout. But it began to recur over the next few days, until eventually Rebecca had to stop exercising altogether. Her energy level was also very low, and she was always tired, even after a good night's sleep. She started to take naps in the middle of the day, which was a first for her. She had to quit her soccer team when she no longer had the stamina to make it through a game. She was only 18 years old, but the pain in her body made her feel like an old lady. Rebecca's parents were worried, because Rheumatoid Arthritis runs in their family and they were afraid that is what Rebecca was developing. After several appointments and blood tests with a long string of different doctors, no one could diagnose Rebecca's condition or explain to her why she was in so much pain.

When she came to visit the Tao of Wellness, they were able to diagnose her right away with Parvo, a virus that attacks the joints. She started treatments and saw immediate improvement. After each acupuncture treatment, Rebecca felt instantly improved and little by little, she felt better every day. With a combination of different herbal formulations and a specific diet plan designed by Dr. Mao and Jason, Rebecca can now exercise again and no longer walks with a limp.

Fibromyalgia and Arthritis

Fibromyalgia is a modern disease that causes muscle and connective tissue pain. A patient is diagnosed with fibromyalgia when 11 out of 18 trigger points throughout the body proved tender, and when the symptoms have been recurring for more than three months. Moving the body can be difficult when the pain becomes widespread, and in that state joints can easily become weak or stiff. Fibromyalgia is often associated with sleep disorders and can also be related to Chronic Fatigue Syndrome. Conventional treatments sometimes employ antidepressants and sleep medications to help increase serotonin production in the brain, improve the patient's sleep, and hopefully ease the pain. This approach has had limited success and some patients are reluctant to take antidepressants when they don't suffer from depression.

For the six million fibromyalgia sufferers in the U.S. there is hope in finding relief through appropriate, low-impact exercise like water aerobics or biking. It is crucial to maintain joint strength and flexibility when fighting against this disease. If you have a fibromyalgia diagnosis or if you're in constant pain in many parts of your body, be sure to see an acupuncturist. There are acupuncture and herbal protocols to activate blood flow, alleviate pain, generate fluids, and reduce inflammation to rehabilitate muscles and joints.

Crohn's, Celiac, Leaky Gut, and Arthritis

Chronic arthritic pain accompanied by digestive problems may be due to inflammatory bowel diseases like Crohn's, colitis, or celiac disease. Many people focus on the joint pain and ignore their digestive problems, but a treatment based on an accurate diagnosis of the digestive condition can often lead to relief of the arthritis. Autoimmune conditions like the ones listed above share a common trait with arthritis: inflammation caused by a hyperactive and overacting immune system that has mistakenly attacked the intestines and the joints. Celiac disease causes intestinal inflammation due to an inability to digest gluten, a protein found in wheat, rye, barley and oats. Elimination of gluten from one's diet usually takes care of the inflammation. The link between the intestines and the joints may be due to a mechanism of "leaky gut" in which a breakdown of the protective mucous membrane of the intestinal wall allows antigens, bacteria, and toxins to cross the barrier and enter the bloodstream, causing inflammation.

Conventional drug treatments for Crohn's and colitis may also employ immunosuppressants used for arthritis that subdue the rebellious immunity, but side effects abound and patients are at high risk for kidney disease and infections due to a suppressed immune system. Chinese herbal medicines like radix coptidis, a plant root from which berberine was isolated, has been found to reduce inflammation, inhibit bacteria, and restore barrier function of the intestines.

Flu, Infections, and Arthritis

For some people, the flu or strep throat they caught during the last cold and flu season may seem to linger. The flu symptoms or the sore throat may have subsided, but the muscle and joint pain remained. For certain sufferers, this is the beginning of long years of arthritis pain. Viruses, bacteria, and parasites can all make trouble for your joints.

For example, there are a host of bacterial organisms that infect joints and cause acute and chronic arthritic inflammation. These range from the more common streptococcus and staphylococcus bacteria to the more obscure Brucella, Pseudomonas, and Borrelia burgdorferi (Lyme disease). Anyone can get infectious arthritis but those most susceptible include people with weakened immunity— children and the elderly, pregnant women, alcoholics, and drug addicts. Patients with diabetes, heart valve defects, kidney disease, AIDS, cancer, or those on steroid or immunosuppressant medications are also at a higher risk. Moreover, working or living in close quarters with farm animals or ingesting contaminated food can also subject one to infectious arthritis. The good news is that by identifying the cause and treating patients accordingly, such as with antibacterial or antiviral medications, permanent relief can often be obtained. Infectious arthritis does not pass from one person to another. If you've had similar onset history with your arthritis you may want to talk to your healthcare practitioner about the possibility of infection as the cause of your condition and seek appropriate treatment.

We recommend natural antimicrobial herbs and nutritional therapy to inhibit infection, acupuncture to support and modulate immune functions, and probiotics to restore intestinal flora.

Reiter's Syndrome—Reactive Arthritis

Sometimes long after the invasion of a bacteria or virus, the cell fragments of the invading microbes can trigger your immune system, creating a cascade of inflammatory reactions that result in arthritis. This is called reactive arthritis, and one example of this is called Reiter's syndrome. Symptoms of Reiter's syndrome include inflammation of the eyes, urethra, skin, and joints, caused by a history of infection that may include sexually transmitted diseases, salmonella, or food poisoning. Because of the widespread, seemingly unconnected symptoms and signs, it is often misdiagnosed. Chinese medicine is well suited to the effective management of Reiter's syndrome because the symptom pattern of the disease has long been recognized by Chinese medicine and the recommended treatment involves detoxification to rid the pathogen and its fragments, reduce inflammation, and increase circulation for healing. This has been accomplished with acupuncture, herbal and nutritional therapies, and Tai Chi.

Frozen Shoulder—Adhesive Capsulitis

Frozen shoulder is a common condition for patients between 40 and 50 years of age. Sometimes it begins with a seemingly minor injury, such as when you reach into the backseat of your car to fetch something and feel a sharp pain in your shoulder. Or you may wake up one day and feel a little stiff, with pain in your shoulder that progressively gets worse, with a range of motion that becomes more restricted over time. This condition is sometimes called frozen shoulder, and is the result of inflammation in the joint capsule, which then affects ligaments that hold the shoulder bones to each other, vastly restricting movement of the arm. The unfortunate side effect is that, because of the shoulder pain, patients tend to stop using the arm. The lack of use leads to more stiffness and even less range of motion. Therefore, exercise and physical therapy for the affected area must be an essential part of a comprehensive treatment program, including acupuncture, which has been shown to be effective for relief of frozen shoulder.

Arthritis in Chinese Medicine – Painful Obstruction

"If there's pain, there's obstruction."
Yellow Emperor's Classic of Medicine

Chinese medicine categorizes joint disorders as Painful Obstruction, also referred to as Bi (pronounced "bee"). There are a variety of disease factors that can cause arthritis, according to Chinese medicine. These include colds invading the joints, pathogenic wind disturbing the joints, dampness congealing in the joints, and heat scorching the joints. Correspondingly, Chinese medicine categorizes arthritic conditions into four types based on their symptom presentation: Cold, Wind, Damp, and Heat types. Two or three can often present at the same time as a combined syndrome.

Chinese medicine has long recognized that invading pathogens such as viruses, bacteria, fungi, or even plain cold air can enter the body and cause obstruction of the normal circulation of energy and body fluids. This is experienced as pain, soreness, numbness, and heaviness in the joints and limbs. Cold, damp, windy weather frequently accompany the onset of the illness in susceptible people and explains why some can sense weather changes as pain and soreness in their joints and bones.

If not treated in a timely fashion, Painful Obstruction, or Bi, can lead to joint or connective tissue weakness. At that point, there will be substantial blockages keeping nutrients from reaching their destination and these tissues will wither and atrophy. Tendons and muscles will shrink or lose strength to the point of appearing thin and flabby. Acting on those initial symptoms of pain and soreness is crucial for joint health and longevity.

The following pages describe the picture of the different types of arthritis, according to Chinese medicine.

Wind Bi Arthritis

Chinese medicine sees an attack of pathogenic Wind as a condition where pain starts acutely, when pain stops and starts, or when it constantly changes locations, much like the actual wind. This usually occurs in the elbows, wrists, knees, and ankles. Joint movement can be limited or accompanied by spasms. There may also be fever or chills because Wind arthritis is typical in those who get colds or flus often. This is indicative of a weaker immune system. Wind arthritis can often combine with the other three types of Painful Obstruction: Damp, Cold, and Heat. "Pathogenic Wind" is Chinese medicine's way of perceiving bacteria and viruses.

The best way to expel these invaders at the surface of your body is with diaphoresis, or sweating. Certain herbal teas or topical oils do this very well. Try boiling and drinking a tea made of one or more of the following: scallions, Chinese basil, mint, ginger, or cinnamon. After drinking the hot tea, bundle up or get under the covers in bed to perspire. Tonic Oil is a wonderful topical treatment for Wind arthritis. It has wintergreen, menthol, sesame, peppermint, and fennel oils to penetrate the body and restore movement to painful joints. You can also put it in your bath. We recommend that you avoid sugar, alcohol, smoking, caffeine, shellfish, and over-exertion. These would provide additional toxins and challenges to an already burdened immune system. See the Appendix for a diet protocol specifically for Wind Bi, and the Resources section for more information on Tonic Oil.

Stephanie's Story

Several years ago, Stephanie came into our office with acute pain in her neck, shoulders, elbows, knees, and back. At the outset she felt she had caught the flu with the usual accompanying body ache but instead of gradually fading away, her pain only grew as time went on. She felt increasing pain in her neck that would shift locations in the mornings to include her elbow or her knees. Stephanie saw her internist who initially advised over the counter pain relievers like Motrin and Advil, and when the pain only got worse he switched her to a prescription anti-inflammatory medication. Her pain did not get better and continued to shift from one joint to another. She struggled to cope with the pain for three weeks without any relief before she came to our office.

We diagnosed her as suffering from Wind Bi arthritis and immediately treated her with acupuncture and cupping, along with vigorous massage to stimulate energy, increase blood flow, and induce sweating. We also sent her home with a customized herbal formula to help support her immunity and fight off the invading pathogen that was the cause of her arthritic pain. We asked her to take a hot bath with tonic oil. That night after the bath she sweated profusely, and per our instructions, she drank plenty of water to keep herself adequately hydrated. The very next morning her pain had drastically decreased. She came in for a follow-up treatment three days later and woke up the next morning with her pains completely subsided. It has not returned since.

Cold Bi Arthritis

Joints with Cold Bi arthritis have pain that's fixed and sharp. This is due to cold, which constricts the blood vessels and tissues. Cold arthritis is alleviated with warm compresses, which help to restore circulation to the affected areas. When ice is applied, the pain will only increase because of further contraction of the tissues. Those susceptible to Cold Bi arthritis usually have a pale complexion and tend to feel chilled. Moxibustion is very effective for Cold Bi arthritis. This is a modality of Chinese medicine where an herb called mugwort is burned to heat an area of the body, or specific acupoints, to restore proper circulation. If this is inconvenient, simply spray mugwort essence on the skin and cover with a warm compress, liniment, or heating pad will also provide some relief.

Other practical solutions include going outside for regular sunshine or drinking warming herbal teas like ginger, cinnamon, and scallion. Winter Tea has many herbs to warm the body, expel cold, and support Kidney function. According to Chinese medicine, the Kidney-Adrenal Network is seen as the body's natural "furnace." We recommend to our patients with Cold Bi arthritis to eat more warming foods, such as green onions, cardamom, mustard, fennel, and horseradish. You'll want to avoid cold and damp environments, raw foods, and icy cold beverages. An effective liniment for topical massage can be made by combining any vegetable or seed oil with freshly ground ginger, garlic, scallion, or cinnamon. See the Resources section for more information on mugwort spray, and the Appendix for more information on the Winter Tea and for a complete diet protocol specifically for Cold Bi.

Sam's Story

As an avid fisherman, Sam has fished all over the world, but one of his favorite pastimes was ice fishing on the Lakes of Minnesota in the dead of winter, an experience he shared with his father while growing up. When Sam came to us he had been suffering from osteoarthritis in his ankles, knee and hip for about five years. He was 49 years old at the time. Our initial consultation revealed that the onset of his arthritis had been about two months after his last ice fishing trip, during which he had suffered frostbite from that week's particularly cold weather. His pain was sharp and consistent in both ankles, his right knee, and his left hip, and had not let up since it began. He had taken many painkillers, anti-inflammatory medications, and even steroids without any relief. The x-ray showed diminished cartilage and his orthopedist was recommending surgery. Sam was opposed to surgery, and came to us out of desperation.

We diagnosed Sam with Cold Bi arthritis and put him on a diet and herbal protocol specific for his condition. He was also treated with weekly acupuncture along with infrared sauna to get rid of the cold. Before he used the sauna we had him take niacin and vitamin B3 to dilate his capillaries and create a warm flushing. We also recommended that Sam take a course of supplements, including vitamin E, fish oil, and MSM, and add hot spices like chili peppers, ginger, and turmeric to his daily diet. Every time Sam came out of the sauna his pain would be substantially diminished.

About four months into his weekly treatments Sam was experiencing almost full relief of his pain and was planning another fishing trip. This time I recommended that he avoid the cold, skip the ice fishing, and go marlin fishing in Baja, Mexico instead!

The Healing Power of Infrared Sauna

When using saunas for treatment, far-infrared saunas are preferable, especially for Cold arthritis because of the warmth of the therapy. But anyone suffering from painful, tight joints will likely see immediate relief. Far-infrared light waves mimic the energetic frequencies of healthy cells and work by breaking the chemical bonds between our body's cells and those of toxic waste products, which are then carried out of the body. The sweat produced by using infrared saunas contains more toxins than what would normally be produced by sweating in a traditional hot room sauna. Heavy metals, such as mercury and aluminum, cholesterol, fat-soluble toxins, sulfuric acid, sodium, ammonia, and uric acid, have been detected in the sweat from a far-infrared sauna treatment. Certain sauna designs allow the head to avoid exposure, permitting people with high blood pressure to benefit as well. Arthritis sufferers can enhance their healing by removing these toxic accumulations, which will allow nourishment to reach the joints quicker and carry away any metabolic waste from your joints. If you aren't sensitive to the "flushing" properties of Niacin, take 100 milligrams about 15 minutes beforehand to enhance the toxin-removing effects of the infrared sauna by stimulating and expanding the small blood vessels.

Damp Bi Arthritis

When moisture from the environment enters your body, you may experience Damp arthritic pain, which presents as numb, heavy, and sore sensations in the joints. These feelings are typically worse during cloudy, rainy days, or wet conditions. This Dampness thickens the bodily fluids and disrupts normal circulation. Those with Damp Bi arthritis may also suffer from sluggishness, mental fog, bloating, or obesity. In Chinese medicine, the stomach, spleen, and pancreas are responsible for the transformation and transportation of the food and beverages we consume, which results in proper digestion under normal circumstances. However, when these processes slow down, our metabolism can weaken to the point that fluid builds up in the tissues. The easiest way to see this is on your tongue. If your tongue is larger than normal or swollen, you may notice teeth marks on the sides. This indicates that your fluid metabolism is sluggish and Dampness may be getting in the way of your optimal health. In Chinese Medicine, we say, "As in nature so is within." In this case, Dampness encourages mold and fungus in nature and within the body ecology dampness hosts yeast, bacteria, fungus, and parasites.

Tea blends containing nutmeg, corn silk, tangerine peel, barley, and green tea also offer simple ways to carry Dampness from the body. Frankincense resin, also known as Boswellia extract, is fantastic for this type of arthritis. It has a warm property, which in combination with its ability to thin and move the blood, makes it ideal for pain relief and relaxation of muscle tissues. It can also reduce swelling and help generate tissue in the joints after overuse or injury. Foods like millet, celery, cucumber, and brown rice break up sticky bodily fluids and produce new fluids to restore proper metabolism. Remember to avoid wheat, dairy, sugar, cold and raw food, greasy and fried foods, and damp environments as all of these can make it worse for arthritis. See the Appendix for a complete diet protocol specifically for Damp Bi.

Jerry's Story

I knew before I met Jerry that he and his wife had been dealing with water damage in their home for over two years because his wife was a long-time patient of mine. The water pipe that burst on the second floor of their home was repaired, but the water damage was extensive, and affected many rooms in the house, including the master bedroom on the first floor. They ripped up and replaced the carpeting and repaired whatever they could see. Several months after the initial water damage, Jerry developed a cough that wouldn't go away for more than a month. He went to see his medical doctor, who thought Jerry had developed bronchitis and prescribed antibiotics. But Jerry continued to cough, and soon he had also developed debilitating pains in his wrists and fingers to the point where he was no long able to type, which had been a critical part of his work performance.

He took ibuprofen to deal with the pain, but the relief lasted a few hours at best and always got worse at night and in the morning. After our initial examination, we diagnosed Jerry with Damp Bi, as he also exhibited many digestive problems, including bloating, gas, and frequent loose bowel movements. We also suspected mold exposure might be causing his immune system to react. Jerry was put on the Detox Diet (see Appendix) we often recommend for Damp Bi arthritis. He also began a treatment course of twice-a-week acupuncture and massage treatments, along with customized herbal formulations and supplements that included digestive enzymes, probiotics, and Boswellia.

I was concerned that possible mold exposure had caused his Damp Bi arthritis, so I referred him to a mold inspector. After air samples came back showing extremely high levels of mold spores, the inspector broke into the master bedroom wall and discovered an entire wall covered with black mold. Jerry and his wife moved out for the duration of the mold abatement and drywall replacement. After five months of treatment and repair on his home, Jerry's arthritis went away completely and never returned. His digestion also normalized.

Heat Bi Arthritis

When one of the other pathogens (Wind, Cold, Damp) is left untreated it will stagnate inside the body, eventually reaching the point
where it creates friction, heat, and inflammation. However, acute
situations like trauma, autoimmune reactions, or infection may also
present similarly. Heat Bi arthritis manifests with joint pain, local
redness, and swelling. If the swelling or deformity is severe it may
limit your ability to move the affected joints. Fever and thirst are
also issues associated with Heat Bi arthritis. Gout is frequently cat-
egorized as a Heat type of joint pain. Simple teas made of mint and
turmeric can cool tissues internally and restore proper blood flow.
Stinging nettle has been shown to reduce the pain and inflammation of arthritis. Nettle can cool tissues and clear toxic buildup, and it
can also be used topically or prepared for internal use in teas, soups,
and extracts.

Another simple topical treatment involves applying a poultice of
crushed dandelion greens every two hours. Smash the leaves in a
mortar and pestle and apply under a cloth. *Tonic Oil* (see Appendix), a formula containing wintergreen, menthol, and peppermint,
is a wonderful way to cool the tissues and penetrate the skin to restore circulation and alleviate pain. Fresh fruits and vegetables are
mostly cooling in nature and are supportive for Heat Bi arthritis. Try
to avoid alcohol, spicy foods, sugar, smoking, stress, and nightshade
vegetables like tomatoes, potatoes, eggplant, and bell peppers, as all
of these promote inflammation and pain. See the Appendix for a
complete diet protocol specifically for Heat Bi.

Patrick's Story

Patrick, Jason's father-in-law, recently went to a rural area of India and, unfortunately, came back with a rare mosquito-borne viral infection called Chikungunya. The disease starts off like a standard bout of flu, but threatens those who contract it with potentially life-long debilitating arthritis. His started similarly, with several symptoms of Heat arthritis, including a high fever, weakness, and joints that became swollen, red, and painful to touch or use. This made the simple process of getting out of bed in the morning a challenge for him, let alone completing his standard exercise routine or going to work and living his life. He was very used to good health and plentiful strength, so this change came as quite a shock. He said his knees, hands, and feet felt as if they were filled with broken glass. Western medicine had nothing to offer as a solution for his condition, because Chikengunya is not well understood by that mode of treatment. Ibuprofen gave him some much-needed pain reduction, but he knew that wasn't going to fix the problem. His problem fit easily into the Heat Bi arthritis type of Painful Obstruction. The treatment we gave him, consisting of Chinese herbal medicine, acupuncture, a low-impact exercise program, and nutritional guidance, followed the recommendations for that category. This meant temporarily stopping his daily cup of coffee and glass of wine, due to their tendency to exacerbate pain and inflammation. At the time of this writing, about four months after first contracting the illness, his condition is all but completely healed. The only symptom left is a very mild discomfort in his hands.

Energy & Blood Depletion

Energy and blood are necessary for every part of the body, including the joints, to thrive. Transporting these resources to the joints requires extra work because the joint is a closed system. Without these supplies, tissues can decay and result in joint pain. Women lose additional blood and energy every month when menstruating, which could explain why both osteoporosis and arthritis are more prevalent in women. Other common causes of this depletion are excessive physical or mental work; excessive sex; an exposure to certain toxins, including alcohol, cigarettes, caffeine, and recreational or pharmaceutical drugs; chronic disease; lack of sleep; a poor diet, including processed foods, fried foods, and excessive sugar and fat; chronic stress; and trauma. Aging itself is responsible for a loss of these nutrients and energetic resources, though at a much steadier pace than the more acute causes mentioned. The best way to avoid losing this precious fuel is to live moderately, minimize overexertion and stress, and incorporate a balanced diet and exercise routine. If this sounds easier said than done, don't worry. While it's commendable to change your entire life in one day, most people need to make these changes gradually over time. To replenish this lost energy, we recommend to our patients an herbal protein supplement called *High Performance*, which contains herbs like Chinese yam, lotus seed, and ginseng with brown rice in an easily digestible formula that can help rebuild lost energy and blood, and also keep your body and joints going strong. See the Appendix for more information on the herbs found in *High Performance* and for a complete diet protocol specifically for energy and blood depletion.

Chapter Two:
Diet and Nutrition

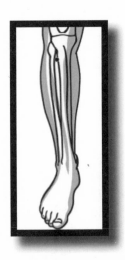

Every day we are given several opportunities to replenish our energy when we eat. Our taste buds enjoy it, if we eat with friends we can make it a social occasion, and the preparation can become an education in food combining and the science of cooking. When all is plated and ready to enjoy, the food choices we make have an immediate effect on our health. Good food, together with regular exercise and a moderate lifestyle, can regenerate tissues, improve our immune systems, stabilize our mood, reduce excess weight, increase energy, improve sleep, and relieve joint pain.

In Chinese medicine, the healing properties of food, especially when tailored to each person's unique needs, have been the cornerstone of Chinese medical nutrition for thousands of years. In other words, Chinese medicine advocates "eat to live" as opposed to "live to eat." Modern research is confirming the perils of the "live to eat" lifestyle, as many degenerative diseases have been linked to the typical American diet, which is typically high in fat, animal protein, refined carbohydrates, sugar, artificial flavoring and coloring, and preservatives. However, exciting discoveries of functional foods, those that possess healthful properties, have validated the "eat to live" model of Chinese medical nutrition.

Here are some examples of functional foods and their properties:
  • Green tea, black tea, and white tea are full of antioxidants and have been found to have anti-cancer and anti-inflammatory properties.
  • Walnuts contain vitamin B6 for healthy nerve cell communication and may benefit your memory.
  • Cucumber contains ascorbic acids that soothe irritated skin and reduce skin inflammation.
  • Sweet potatoes reduce C-reactive protein, which is a cell-signaling protein that causes inflammation
  • Soy milk may decrease pain and lower the risk of prostate cancer.
  • Chili pepper contains capsaicin that gives food a spicy kick and fights inflammation.

• Foods like salmon, sardines, and tuna are good sources of Omega-3 fatty acids and can reduce inflammation.

Certain common foods are known to aggravate inflammation and pain, and most people with arthritis would benefit from avoiding them. You might notice more pain and stiffness in your joints the morning after a dinner of pasta with tomato sauce, grilled eggplants, and bell peppers with a side of roasted potatoes. Why? Because these foods, excluding the pasta, belong to a plant family called night-shades that contain the alkaloid solanine. While it isn't terribly toxic, solanine is known to elicit inflammatory responses in individuals with arthritis.

Eat well for your body, for your mind, and for your life!

Less Weight, Less Pain

The majority of Americans today are overweight. More than 68% of the nation, a total of more than 207 million people and two out of every three individuals, are carrying at least 10 extra pounds. Additionally, one out of every three Americans is obese. This means that more than 101 million people are overweight in excess of 30 pounds. These numbers are staggering. All that added weight increases the risk for arthritis. Extra weight is obviously a problem for the weight-bearing joints like the knees and hips, but it can stress almost any joint. Being overweight on top of suffering from arthritis can make exercise more difficult, and a lack of movement makes both the weight and joint problems that much worse.

This downward spiral needs to be broken. What's more, your risk of developing Type II Diabetes rises exponentially if you are overweight, not to mention other serious conditions, including heart disease.

If you need help getting started with your weight loss, consult a nutritionist and a fitness instructor. Tackling 50 or 100 extra pounds can seem impossible, so focus on losing 10 pounds at a time. When you've reached your first 10-pound goal, celebrate and congratulate yourself on a job well done before getting to work on the next 10 pounds. Don't give in to the temptation to weigh yourself more than once per week. Statistics show that success comes quicker to those who focus on how they look and feel, rather than just the number on the scale. Try to make eating and exercising fun. It's hard to keep up a regimen if you're not enjoying yourself.

Be Responsible for Your Health

The majority of the extra body weight plaguing America is entirely self-made. By "self-made," we are not only referring to the hundreds of millions of people making their daily choices at their markets, restaurants, and kitchens, but the actions of our governments and corporations in producing excessive quantities of poor quality, heavily processed, and highly sugared foods. Humans are still hard-wired to eat whatever is in front of us in the hope that we will be prepared for an impending famine. Your body instinctively responds by storing this extra energy away as fat. Food scientists understand this mechanism well and have gradually "super-sized" food portions over the past few decades, resulting in many super-sized bodies.

However, the American famine has yet to come, so the fat keeps piling on. If you're asking yourself how your body got to this point, blaming yourself, your family, or the television ads won't help you at all. Take responsibility for your health by surrendering any desire to place blame on anyone, including yourself, and get to work on the steps that will erase the excess weight. This includes working with your health team to devise a customized eating plan, exercise routine, and a list of practical, attainable goals. Simple things to try right away include eating out less often, reading labels on the food you buy, and exercising 30 minutes each day. If you recognize that an emotional response is getting in the way of small changes like these, working with a therapist or life coach will bring significant relief and help free you to do the work needed to better your life.

You Are What You Are Made Of

Chinese medical nutrition emphasizes eating foods that directly support organs or tissues in need of help. Examples include eating eggs to support fertility, fruit and vegetable peels to nourish the skin, and in the case of degrading cartilage in our joints, to consume gristle to strengthen our cartilage. We realize that a bowl full of gristle may not be an appetizing idea. But the popular supplements for joint support, Glucosamine and Chondroitin Sulfate, are both derived from similar tissues from other animals, specifically shellfish exoskeleton and cow cartilage. For the non-vegetarian crowd, consuming 4 oz. of lean red meat twice weekly can also be part of a regime to support cartilage production and repair. However, recipes that include bone marrow or tendon can be tasty, like using cow or sheep bones for stock. We also recommend eating the cartilage at the end of chicken bones. Other foods that aid in cartilage production that are more easily found include eggs, black beans, avocado, and grapes.

Moderation is Key to Health and Healing

Sometimes when people are given a list of foods to avoid in their diet, they react in disbelief, as if it were impossible to eat less sugar or to cut out something like coffee, which has become a daily ritual for millions of people. Before you respond negatively, remember that the plan your acupuncturist gives you has been customized for your particular joint imbalance. If you do have certain unhealthy habits, or strong addictions to certain foods or flavors, going cold turkey might not be the best remedy. It may be better to gradually step down, moving from four cups of coffee per day to two cups and then to a single cup, rather than completely eliminating it right away. Losing weight is another great example of how a gradual, step-by-step process of change may be more beneficial than one big leap.

Most people know what they shouldn't be eating. But when you turn cookies into an enemy or cut out sweets completely, it's easy to develop a love/hate relationship with food, which will not be beneficial to you in the long run. Moderation is the key. The most important part is making modifications to the things we eat every day. If you feel you can cut things out completely right away, go for it. But if you despair at the idea of sipping water when everyone else at the birthday party is clinking their wine glasses around you, then it may be all right to allow yourself in a little wine, just so long as it isn't a regular part of your week. This is about practicing healthy new behaviors and relationships with your food. Most of the time remember to focus on eating to live, but every once in awhile it's perfectly alright to live to eat. Work with your acupuncturist or nutritionist to find the diet that's right for you.

Cold Foods Are Too Cold for Your Body

Think about this fact: your body temperature is 98.6 degrees Fahrenheit. Room temperature is generally around 73 degrees. Food taken directly from the fridge is usually less than 50 degrees, depending on the setting. Ice-cold beverages and frozen desserts are often below 32 degrees. Now, imagine putting cold or icy foods or beverages down your esophagus and into your stomach that has a temperature differential of 50 degrees or more. What do you think would happen to your body? Not only does it have to work quickly to warm up the food to body temperature, but in the interim the blood vessels in the lining of your esophagus and stomach constrict in response to the cold injury, diminishing the flow of oxygen and nutrients to them. Over time the lining weakens, predisposing you to erosion of the lining, ulcers, and even polyps. In order to heal your body and joints, you need your digestion to function at peak efficiency, so that it can assist your body in assimilating nutrients from food and herbs. Eat food and drink beverages at room or body temperature and your body will thank you for it.

Raw Food is Not For Everyone

People with normal immune systems can handle uncooked fruits, vegetables, and meat just fine. But some people have a genetic predisposition to sensitive immune and digestive systems, which makes consuming uncooked foods more difficult, since raw foods have more bacteria and fungi on them. Did you know that cooking was originally used to kill microorganisms and sterilize food? Organic foods are prone to hosting even more microbes than non-organic foods because no pesticides have been used on them. So while we advocate organic food to our patients, we also advise them to wash and cook it well. Raw foods, with all the foreign life living on them, can be seen as spoiled food by your immune system. When these foreign entities are introduced into your body, your immune system can spring into action by producing mucus to trap and flush out these invaders. If this response is excessive, then the mucus can also get in the way of proper digestion.

According to Chinese medicine, raw foods are considered cold in nature. We're warm-blooded creatures, and our digestive and metabolic processes are dependent on warmth to carry out their functions, which include breaking down food, releasing enzymes, and transporting food down the digestive tract. This digestive Fire is best supported by foods that are lightly cooked. Some feel that cooking destroys the nutrients in food, and while overcooking foods will certainly "kill" them in this way, a light cooking will simply open the cell walls, giving us easier access to these nutrients without requiring our bodies to cook the food internally. For example, the antioxidant lycopene in tomatoes isn't released until the tomato is cooked.

The best way to make sure your fruits and vegetables are being cooked properly is to watch for the color to become brighter. When this is the case, take it off the stove. If the color has gone away then you've overshot optimal cooking time. Most fruits and vegetables only need a couple minutes of cooking.

Be a Host to Good Guests Only

Mucus membranes secret mucus and are present all throughout your body. They line your respiratory system in the nose, throat, and lungs. They also line the digestive tract from mouth to anus. In women they're present in the vagina. There is also mucus production in other areas, such as the urinary tract, ears, and eyes. And anywhere there is moisture and mucus, there is potential for bacterial and fungal growth. These bacteria can help us or hurt us. It's best when there is a balance between the two, because positive bacteria act as part of our immune system, fighting off overgrowth of nearby negative bacteria and fungi as well as other pathogens from outside our body. It's when these good bacteria dwindle that their negative neighbors steal more room and resources to multiply and challenge our tissues and immune function.

Candida is the most common fungal overgrowth, and is typically found in the genitals and the digestive and urinary systems. Candida and many other types of fungi and bacteria can migrate to our joints as well, causing infection and a weakened joint metabolism. This can either set the stage for arthritis or worsen any joint pain that's already present. Control this fungus by taking a probiotic supplement with at least one billion active beneficial, bacterial cultures to rebalance the intestinal flora. Also, try to avoid foods like wheat, sugar, alcohol, and dairy that can serve as fuel for a growing fungus or bacteria. Proper gut flora can also be supported with naturally fermented foods like yogurt, miso (fermented soybean paste that's great in soups), tempeh, natto (whole fermented soybeans), and kimchi (Korean fermented cabbage that's sour, spicy, and tasty). Candida and other overgrowths can also get in the way of weight loss and other chronic diseases, so do yourself a big favor and be a host to good guests only.

Your Body Clock for Optimum Digestion

Breakfast is the most important meal because your body's daily clock, which is observed in both Chinese medicine and biological science as the circadian rhythm, has our digestive organs literally "waking up" not long after we do. Chinese medicine observed that our stomach is most active from 7 – 9 o'clock in the morning. Digestion and metabolic activities will slow down if not given work to do soon after waking up.

These processes will also be burdened by eating too close to bedtime. The only thing you should be doing while sleeping is, well, sleeping. Not much digesting should happen while you're asleep, because this is the time of day your body rests and therefore consumes little. This slows the metabolism and packs on extra weight. You should finish eating at least three hours before you plan to go to sleep. But while you're awake, try to eat something once every three hours. A simple meal schedule would be something like: 6am, 9am, 12pm, 3pm, 6pm. Eating small meals, consistently throughout the day, is the proper way to train your metabolism. If you are trying to lose weight, skipping meals will work against you by slowing your metabolism. If you are underweight, limiting yourself to three meals a day may not cut it. The ideal is an evenly-paced digestion.

You should think of the digestive system like a campfire; you can easily put out the fire by both under- or over-feeding it. Small twigs won't be enough to keep a fire big enough to keep you warm, and dumping a trashcan full of wood on a small fire will put it out as well. Slow and steady is the key. Food choice and preparation are very important, but people often overlook the value of quantity and timing in their diet plans.

Your Stomach Doesn't Have Teeth

Multitasking is the collective way of life these days. We have trained ourselves to do many things at once, and we're often rewarded for how well we can juggle the different parts of our lives. But when it comes time have a meal, the only thing you should be focusing on is eating. Socializing is generally no problem, but loud music, television, computers, books, and other distractions like driving or working can make digesting more difficult. This can quickly slow down your metabolism and make optimizing your weight more challenging. After just a few days of eating in a more relaxed environment, you may find you have less gas and have a better idea of when you've had enough food. It's easy to miss signals from your body that tell you when you feel satisfied or full if there are a dozen other things going on in your environment or your mind.

Chewing your food completely will help to properly start your digestion. Digestion starts in the mouth, and contrary to what some people may believe, your stomach can't make up the difference for food that hasn't been chewed well. The stomach doesn't have teeth, so do your tummy a favor and break up the food completely before you send it down to be digested. When food is chewed well, the flavors are enhanced, and you may soon find that you need less salt or other spices when you fully experience the food and not just what you put on top of it. Chewing slowly and steadily is also helpful in relaxing the rest of the body while eating.

Fresh Foods, Clean Hands

Wash your hands and wash your food before every meal. This may seem like a no-brainer, but some simple tasks don't seem obvious until after you get sick. But keeping pathogens out of your body can be simple, as unwashed hands and food are two of the top ways in which you ingest these invaders. Kids frequently get sick because they don't wash their hands and they pass germs back and forth with other kids while at school or day care. Restaurant workers pass infectious diseases like hepatitis A to patrons by not following hygienic requirements, and E. Coli outbreaks resulting from contaminated produce are becoming commonplace. To avoid bringing harmful contaminants into your food supply, be aware of your food handling process. Keep two separate cutting boards in your kitchen, one for uncooked meats and the other for fresh produce or cooked foods. Avoid cross contamination between the two cutting boards and always wash your hands with soap after handling raw meats. Be sure to cook everything and refrain from eating raw foods whenever possible.

The Good and Bad of Alcohol

Chinese medicine has regularly used alcohol as a carrier of herbal remedies in tincture form. And in some cases, an arthritis patient may actually benefit from a nightly shot of herbal liqueur. But for most people, this is not the case, and everyone should consult their physician before considering alcohol as part of their arthritis regiment. The types of alcohol used in making tinctures and in therapeutic shots are pure stills. Clear spirits like vodka are clean and have fewer impurities than beer and wine, which are full of sulfites. Sulfite residue can easily get stuck in the joints and make pain or stiffness much worse. Traditionally, herb liqueur is made by infusing select herbs into bottles of high-proof alcohol and then aging the tincture for several months. Small shots taken before bedtime can improve circulation and warm the joints. Try to avoid drinking during the day, especially before driving, and be sure to check your liver functions regularly. You should stop if your body shows any adverse reactions. Pregnant women and people who have alcohol addictions should absolutely refrain from it and seek out a different remedy among the ones outlined in this book.

Cut Coffee, Try Tea Instead

Coffee is one of the largest commodities on the global market. Our planet is practically hard-wired to wake up with a cup or two (or three!) of caffeine every day. But coffee has high levels of caffeine and acids and should generally be avoided by arthritis sufferers. Drinking caffeinated beverages while suffering from painful arthritis is like adding fuel to the fire, making the pain that much worse.

Try a green, white or black tea instead. The polyphenols in tea have been shown to be protective against arthritis and good for reducing inflammation. For thousands of years, tea has been used as a healing agent by many cultures around the world. That's because green tea is among the most potent sources of antioxidants and includes catechins, substances that inhibit the activity of cartilage-degrading enzymes. If you can learn to kick the coffee habit and switch to tea, your joints will thank you.

More Sugar Leads to More Pain

Sugar in its natural form is the food that each of our cells requires for production of ATP. ATP stands for adenosine triphosphate and it is the energy we release in our cells that allows our bodies to do everything. Refined sugars, on the other hand, are pro-inflammatory substances which can make pain and joint inflammation worse. But it can be difficult to know which is which. Put simply, if the sugar is in a whole food like fruit or milk then there is much less concern for a spike in your blood sugar levels. This is because the sugar is bound to the whole food's protein or fiber counterpart, essentially time releasing the sugar into our bloodstream and avoiding an excessive sugar dump into our system. On the other hand, almost anything that's meant to sweeten your food has been refined to some degree. Two notable exceptions would be Stevia leaf and raw honey, but even these should be used in moderation.

Cane sugar, agave syrup, brown rice syrup, fructose, brown sugar, turbinado sugar, sucrose, and lactose are all refined sugars and should be avoided if you want less pain and inflammation. One study directly links fructose consumption in juice and soda with an increased risk of gout. So if you need a little extra sweetness but want to avoid aggravating your pain, reach for a little raw honey or Stevia rather than pure sugar.

Go for the Shell but Leave the Flesh

Shellfish are a common source of food allergies, and can also be the cause of severe food poisoning. But the allergic reaction and the food poisoning happen for very different reasons. The allergy is due to an imbalance within a person's immune system. Food poisoning occurs because the shellfish has not been cooked properly.

People can be affected by one or both classes of shellfish. Mollusks, like clams and oysters, have the characteristic double shell. Crustaceans, like shrimp, lobster, and crab, have an exoskeleton that keeps the outside of their body hard and protected. But it's not the shell or exoskeleton that causes the allergic reaction. It's the fleshy meat itself that's responsible. It should be noted that the popular arthritis supplement glucosamine is made of crustacean exoskeleton. A reputable glucosamine company will not have mixed the animal's flesh in with the shell, so arthritis sufferers with a shellfish allergy should be able to take glucosamine without a problem.

Avoid the Nightshades

Chinese medicine views many types of pain as inflammation, and eating certain common foods can be like adding fuel to the fire, making inflammatory pain worse. The nightshade family of vegetables can stimulate an inflammatory reaction in the body when you eat them. Nightshades include potatoes, tomatoes, eggplant, and bell peppers. Its most famous cousin, belladonna, is a highly toxic plant that was thought to be responsible for several mysterious deaths in Medieval Europe. Modern research has discovered the culprit—Solanine, an alkaloid that irritates the immune system and leads to the inflammatory response. Clinically, we've found that small amounts of these foods are tolerated by patients with mild cases of arthritis. This includes a few pieces of sun-dried tomatoes, a couple small potatoes, or a slice or two of eggplant. One study showed that lutein, an antioxidant found in tomatoes, might protect against osteoarthritis. However, during active disease flare-ups it is advisable to stay away from the nightshades completely until after it calms down.

Be Aware of Acids: Oxalic and Uric Acids

An acidic environment can sometimes make pain worse through-out your whole body. Foods rich in oxalic acid – spinach, rhubarb, chives, parsley, and chard – can potentially combine with minerals in the body to form stones that lodge in the kidney, gall bladder, or the joints. Gout-like pain can be due to oxalic acid buildup, but true gout is due to excessive uric acid. But gout isn't the only problem that can result from too much uric acid. It can lead to diabetes and cardiovascular disease. Excess uric acid in the bloodstream comes as a result of consuming too much fructose (high amounts of which are found in fruit juices, dried fruits, and refined table sugar), meat, and rich foods. Other things like fried and greasy foods, wheat, and dairy can also affect the inflammatory process. Avoiding these pro-inflammatory acids may help reduce pain in your joints.

The Good Acids: Fatty Acids Help Fight Inflammation

Nuts and seeds like walnuts, almonds and sesame seeds contain rich supplies of omega-3 fatty acids, which assist in reducing inflammation in the body. Just a handful of nuts and seeds every day can help improve circulation, build muscle tone, and benefit the joints.

Arginine is especially abundant in nuts and seeds. It is a nonessential amino acid, a substance our bodies produce in the liver and deplete during times of stress. Arginine is helpful in fighting heart disease, infertility, and high blood pressure as well as facilitating the healing process. Other benefits of nuts and seeds include increasing cognitive function, preventing diabetes, lowering cholesterol and reducing the risk of heart diseases. Eat a handful every and feel it soothe your inflammation.

The Perils of Soda Pop

Dentists have been warning us for years that soft drinks increase cavities and wear down your tooth enamel due to their sugar and acidity. Average soft drinks have a pH level of 2.8-4. It has been determined that any pH of 5.5 or below is bad for the tooth enamel, so it comes as no surprise that just about all sodas are bad for your teeth. And if it's bad for your teeth, it's a safe bet that it's also bad for your bones and joints.

You may feel "safe" because you're drinking the diet kind and avoiding calories so you won't put on weight. The bad news is that studies have shown that diet soft drinks are associated with an increased risk of heart disease and stroke. But calories aren't the only drawback in colas and other carbonated beverages—they can deplete the calcium in your bones because they contain phosphoric acid, which makes calcium pass out of your system in your urine. For arthritic patients who have an increased risk of osteoporosis, it's even more critical that you avoid soft drinks. If you crave a bubbly refreshment, drink carbonated mineral water and add a slice of lemon!

Good Fats vs. Bad Fats

Not all fats are equal when it comes to arthritis. The bad fats will increase the inflammation in your joints, or worse, clog up your arteries and give you diabetes. Good fats, on the other hand, can reduce your inflammation and even protect you from heart disease.

There are two main types of harmful fats: saturated and trans fats. Saturated fats mainly come from animal sources and include red meat, butter, and lard. Trans fats are mostly man-made fats. They are created by hydrogenation, the process of adding hydrogen to fats to increase shelf life and make foods less likely to spoil or go rancid. Both of these fats increase cholesterol, especially the bad kind (low-density lipoprotein, or LDL), and lower the good kind (high-density lipoprotein, or HDL), all while increasing the inflammatory process in the body. These should always be avoided.

When it comes to beneficial fats, there are two kinds: monounsaturated and polyunsaturated fats. These unsaturated fats mainly come from plant-based and seafood sources, including olive oil, rice bran oil, grape seed oil, walnut oil, hemp seed oil, flax seed oil, and fish oil. The good fats are good for you because they do the opposite of the bad fats; they protect you from heart disease and reduce inflammation. For arthritis sufferers, this is good news.

Tropical Magic for Your Inflammation

Why is arthritis less prevalent in the tropics than in the northern hemisphere? The answer may lie in the abundant tropical fruits consumed by its inhabitants. Researchers have long found beneficial enzymes like papain and bromelain in tropical fruits like papaya and pineapple, respectively. These enzymes assist not only in digestion but also in reducing inflammation. They help by breaking down proteins in the blood that cause inflammation, removing fibrin, the clotting material that prolongs inflammation, and reducing swelling in the areas of inflammation. Other fruits that contain beneficial enzymes are passion fruit, mangos and kiwis.

The next time you're at the market, put some tropical fruits into your cart and start experiencing some tropical magic in your joints. You can also take papain and bromelain in capsules, which are usually available at your local health food store or online. See the Resources section for more information.

Nature's COX-2 Inhibitors

There are two types of enzymes prevalent in the human body called cyclo-oxygenase (COX), or COX-1 and COX-2. The COX-1 enzyme is found in most tissues and is in involved in protecting the stomach lining, ensuring kidney health, and encouraging proper clotting. The COX-2 enzyme on the other hand is a critical component of the inflammation process, but when inflammation gets out of control and results in arthritis or other chronic inflammatory disorders, pain is the consequence. Drugs like Celebrex are prescribed to block COX-2 but have terrifying side effects, like an increased risk of heart disease and strokes. That's where natural COX-2 inhibitors found in our diet and herbs are preferable, because they can help without the side effects. These include turmeric, red grape, rosemary, green tea and bee propolis.

Red Meat Increases Your Risk of Rheumatoid Arthritis

Recently, a team of British researchers found that a diet lacking in fruit, especially varieties high in vitamin C, increases the risk of inflammatory arthritis, a common early warning sign of rheumatoid arthritis, as much as three-fold. Building on this compelling finding, they set out to investigate the association of other dietary habits with the onset of RA. Their results indicate a high level of red meat consumption as an independent risk factor for inflammatory arthritis. Other studies have implicated red meat in increasing risks of cancer, heart disease, and inflammation. If you like to eat red meat, keep it to no more than two times a week in order to keep it from affecting your arthritis. Eat more fish, nuts, and beans instead.

Berry Very Good for Inflammation

When inflammation strikes your body, chemicals, toxins, and harmful enzymes damage tiny blood vessels, causing blood to leak into surrounding tissues. Inflammation also prevents nutrients and oxygen from reaching targeted tissue such as cartilage, ligaments and joints. Anthocyanins, antioxidants found in the pigment of the skin of blueberries, black berries, raspberries and other fruits, protect the body in several ways. First, they neutralize enzymes that destroy connective tissue. Second, their antioxidant capacity prevents oxidants from damaging connective tissue. Finally, they repair damaged proteins in the blood-vessel walls and help reduce allergic and inflammatory reactions. Studies show that anthocyanins possess more potent anti-inflammatory properties than all other flavonoids tested. Add a handful of berries to your meal and have yourself a berry, merry good time!

More than the Symbol for Fertility: Pomegranate

Pomegranate means "apple seeds" in Latin. Long celebrated as a fruit of fertility, abundance, and good luck, pomegranate has been eaten during holidays and celebrations since ancient Hebrew and Greek times. In recent years, pomegranate has been commercially cultivated for its juice. Recent studies have shown that pomegranate has been found to assist in protecting cartilage from the adverse effect of the pro-inflammatory protein interleukin-1b (IL-1b) and the prevention of cartilage degeneration. The IL-1b molecules cause an overproduction of inflammatory compounds and while that is normal in tissue repair, if you suffer from osteoarthritis this excess production can lead to more joint damage and destruction.

The bright red pomegranate seeds can be used as a beautiful garnish, sprinkled in salads or cooked with poultry. It may be good for your fertility and joints, too!

Ginger Works Better Than Drugs

Ginger has a long history, dating back several thousand years in China, of providing both culinary and medicinal use for arthritic pain. Modern research has discovered that it possesses anti-inflammatory properties. One of the therapeutic ingredients, gingerols, as well as other active compounds, has been shown to suppress pro-inflammatory factors like cytokines and chemokines and prevent free radical damage to the joint tissue. Specifically, it has even been shown to work better than drugs for arthritic knees. In a study of patients with rheumatoid arthritis, osteoarthritis, and muscular discomfort, the majority of those who received ginger experienced relief of pain and swelling. Include as much ginger in your diet plan as possible; add ginger to your dishes, make a tea out of fresh ginger root, and take it in capsule form as well.

Curry to the Rescue

Turmeric is a popular cooking spice found in curry that comes from the curcuma plant in the ginger family. It is native to tropical South Asia and has been used in traditional medicines for the treatment of sprains, strains, bruises, and inflammation of the joints. Turmeric is also used for jaundice and other liver ailments, ulcers, parasitic infections, various skin diseases, cold and flu symptoms, as well as for preserving food and promoting digestion. Many studies have been conducted on turmeric and have found it to possess anti-inflammatory and anti-cancer properties. The blood-thinning drug Cumadin was originally extracted from turmeric, so it is also known for its anti-clotting properties. A word of caution: those taking blood thinners should check with their doctors before taking turmeric supplements.

This herb is used primarily for pain, particularly from traumatic injury, as well as pain in the chest, flanks, abdomen, or discomfort related to menstruation. It also calms the emotions and is used to treat anxiety, agitation, and insomnia. Oil of turmeric can be used as a natural insect repellent. You will surely want to add the spice to your cooking to promote healthy circulation. Turmeric can be found fresh in some stores' produce sections and is available as a powder, as a chopped and dried herb, and as a tea, tincture, oil, or poultice.

Cayenne: The Healing Pepper

Throughout the ages, chili peppers have been used for pain relief. In Chinese medicine it has been used to activate blood circulation, "warm up" your body's interior, relieve abdominal pain due to digestive or menstrual disorders, and kill parasites. The powerful heat in cayenne peppers comes from capsaicin, which not only gives food a spicy kick but also fights inflammation. Research shows that it has proven effective in healing pain associated with arthritis, back pain, and nerve pain, as well as greatly improving the condition of psoriasis, especially when applied topically. Capsaicin cream is usually used to relieve pain and itching. Though its ability to reduce a pain-transmitting neurochemical is most effective when applied to the skin, Capsaicin can also be helpful for easing joint stiffness and relieving sore muscles.

However, you may want to skip over this particular pepper if you have red, burning pain in your joints or if you experience heartburn or indigestion. Cayenne and capsaicin are also available in capsule form.

Nature's Collagen: Jellyfish and Sea Cucumbers

Sea cucumbers and jellyfish are found worldwide, and in Asia they are eaten as a delicacy, as they are considered to be food for beauty and longevity. A number of studies found that jellyfish and sea cucumbers contain a rich supply of mucopolysaccharides, chondroitin sulfate, saponins, and fatty acids—nutrients essential for making collagen and cartilage. Besides being good for making your face look younger, as collagen is helpful in maintaining the structural tone of the skin, collagen-rich jellyfish and sea cucumber are also good for your joints.

Chondroitin sulfate is commonly used as an over-the-counter treatment for arthritis pain. Many studies confirmed that the consumption of chondroitin sulfate is effective in reducing arthritis pain in study subjects with moderate to severe arthritis pain. The results of these studies directly link the effectiveness of sea cucumber and jellyfish for treatment of arthritis pain due to the high concentration of chondroitin sulfate.

Both are available fresh or dried in Asian markets. You can also take supplements that contain collagen, like Collagen Boost. See the Resources section for more information.

Keep a Food Journal for a Week

The simple act of putting pen to paper over the course of a week and reviewing it afterward can be very revealing. As you'll see, this journal is not just about food, but also incorporates sleep schedules, exercise, and other markers to see exactly how you spend your day caring for yourself. Generally, five smaller, similarly-sized meals daily (three meals and two snacks) tends to be much easier on the digestion than the three large meals most Americans are used to. Think of your digestion as a small fire. You want to ensure you don't smother the fire with an overabundance of fuel all at once. Gradually feeding the fire smaller pieces at an even pace will keep an even burn going throughout the day. This way, your body will be more able to extract proper nutrients from the foods, herbs, and supplements you give it, thereby giving your body a greater chance to circulate that nourishment to the places it needs to go. Before an initial consultation with any health professional about food or lifestyle choices, fill out at least one week of this journal. Be as detailed as you can and include estimated portion size. See Appendix for a sample food journal.

What Has More Calcium Than Milk and More Iron Than Beef?

The answer is seaweed. There are more than 20 types of edible seaweed being produced and eaten around the world. These seaweeds belong to one of several groups of multicellular algae: red algae, green algae, and brown algae, and most (but not all) are harvested from the sea.

The most popular ones in the U.S. include nori, wakame and kombu. Nori is used as an outer wrap for sushi rolls and is often found in miso soup. Just one sheet of nori has the same amount of omega-3 fatty acids as two whole avocados. Wakame is used in seaweed salad with cucumbers and rice vinegar. It's rich in B vitamins, calcium, magnesium, and trace minerals, which gives it a diuretic property and helps reduce bloating and water retention. Kombu is high in iodine, which is critically important in the production of two key thyroid hormones that control our metabolism. It also contains fucoxanthin in its pigment that may boost production of a protein involved in fat metabolism. Kombu is often boiled and used as stock—the Japanese equivalent of chicken stock. Seaweed is widely available in markets with Asian food aisles, and many health food stores.

Keep Sodium Intake Low for Better Joint Health

Sodium is sometimes implicated in high blood pressure and excluded from the diets of patients with hypertension. It may also be a good idea for people suffering from arthritis to reduce their salt intake. Sodium attracts water molecules and often leads to water retention and swelling in the body. For some people, when this happens around their joints it creates stiffness and pain. Too much sodium in your diet increases the loss of calcium from your body. A 2-year study of postmenopausal women observed increased urinary sodium levels, an indication of high salt intake and increased bone loss in the hips. Try to keep your salt intake low and use herbs and spices in its place for better joint and bone health.

Spice up Your Moves with Cooking Herbs

People who use more herbs and spices seem to be healthier and suffer from fewer diseases, according to studies. Besides making foods tasty and flavorful, herbs and spices can be used as salt substitutes with beneficial results. Many herbs and spices contain antioxidant and anti-inflammatory properties. That list includes garlic, turmeric, ginger, oregano, sage, and clove. The former three are well known for their healing properties whereas the latter three are less so.

Oregano has the highest antioxidant levels of the 39 various types of spices. Although it has gained popularity in more recent times as an anti-bacterial and anti-fungal, oregano has remained as one of the most powerful anti-inflammatory herbs available. Sage has been shown to bring relief for symptoms of arthritis and joint pain. Sage is rich in phenolic acid, flavonoids and antioxidants which all act to protect the body from injury due to bacteria, pollution, and free radicals. Clove is traditionally used a toothache remedy. It contains a powerful anti-inflammatory compound called eugenol that promotes relief beyond toothache to include arthritic pains. So go ahead and sprinkle herbs generously to spice up your moves. See the Appendix for a spice mix recipe.

Power Cereal: Healing Herbs and Whole Grains

In China, breakfast has traditionally been considered the most important meal of the day, so it's no surprise that in the imperial palaces there had long been an emphasis on making breakfast foods full of energizing and healing properties. One of the most popular breakfast options among the palace royals was a nourishing and satisfying hot cereal of 25 herbs, grains, legumes, and seeds for sustained life-force energy, strong bones and joints, healthy digestion, and beautiful hair and skin.

This cereal includes select Chinese herbs like wild yam, fox nut, and poria to promote long life; whole gluten-free grains such as brown rice, black rice, and oats; legumes and beans like lentils, black beans, and mung beans; and nuts and seeds like sesame, lotus, and chestnuts. Cook for a few hours or overnight in a crock pot for a hot delicious cereal. Add seasoning and spices, or sweeten with fresh berries and honey. See the Appendix for recipe.

Keep Gluten from Binding up Your Body

In recent years, more and more gluten-free products have hit the store shelves. If you have been wondering what all the fuss is about, gluten is a protein found in commonly consumed grains, such as wheat, rye, barley, and oats. It is often added in baking to bind the rest of the ingredients together and give the pastry its form and structure. But for the approximately one million people in the United States with Celiac disease, accidental ingestion of gluten can cause serious health consequences, including severe abdominal pain, diarrhea or constipation, fatigue, joint pain, weight loss, or weight gain. Celiac patients are missing the enzyme that allows our bodies to break down gluten, and therefore are intolerant of it. However, there are many others who do not have celiac disease but are still sensitive to gluten. Gluten intolerance and gluten sensitivity are both due to an autoimmune or allergic response that can lead to other inflammatory conditions like arthritis. Many of our patients have experienced substantial relief of their arthritic pain after switching to a diet free of gluten. Try it for a month and see if you find the reprieve others have been experiencing.

Cleanse and Detox for Health and Wellness

Toxins from the environment, as well as those generated internally from infections and inflammation, can trigger your immune system to overreact and create a cascade of ongoing inflammatory responses. Chemicals from everyday encounters include polychlorinated biphenyl (PCBs) from plastics, dioxins from bleached paper products, and artificial colors, flavors, and preservatives in food. These are only a few of the thousands of chemicals that we are exposed to on a regular basis. Studies have shown that many environmental toxins and pollutions are at the root of chronic, degenerative, and inflammatory diseases, including cancer. Add in the fragments of past viral, bacterial, and fungal infections you have encountered, as well as waste products accumulated over many years, and you've got the ingredients of a health breakdown.

But you don't have to be a victim of toxins. Fight back by initiating a cleanse and detox program right at home. Start each day by squeezing a fresh lemon into a glass with 12 oz of warm water and drinking it on an empty stomach. The lemon activates your liver's detoxification process. Throughout the day, drink at least four to six glasses of fresh vegetable juice and broth as a way to supply your body with critical vitamins, minerals, and antioxidants. Eat three high-fiber meals that include brown rice, quinoa, amaranth, leafy green vegetables, seaweed, ground flax seeds, mung beans, and if desired, organic egg whites and poultry. Drink a tea made from herbs like dandelion and peppermint to help excrete toxins from your body. You can stay on this diet for a week and repeat as often as you like. At the Tao of Wellness our medical detox program incorporates, in addition to the diet sessions, dry skin brushing, cupping, lymphatic tuina massage, acupuncture, and infrared sauna treatments along with customized detox herb formulas and supplements to greatly enhance the outcome. Many of our patients with rheumatoid arthritis report at an immediate relief of at least 60% of their pain after participating in the detox program. See the appendix for the Tao of Wellness Detox Diet.

The Healing Power of Fasting

The majority of the waste products found in your body come from the process of eating, not just the food that you eat. On a daily basis, digestion and metabolism generate tremendous amounts of toxins and wastes, some of which can overwhelm your system, leading to pain and inflammation. A simple way to reduce waste overload in your body is to take up fasting. Fasting has been a time-tested healing method since ancient times. In every medical tradition around the world there were written records of fasting for health and relief from illness. Published research found an improvement of arthritis symptoms with fasting. The method is easy, and I suggest choose a light activity day like Sunday on which to practice your fast. Traditional fasting calls for drinking a glass of warm water for every waking hour. I suggest drinking fluids hourly, but substitute at least 4-6 glasses of water with a mix of vegetable juice, vegetable broth, and apple juice. A number of our patients have done this one day a month for many years and have felt more energy, mental clarity and improved skin complexion.

A word of caution on fasting: while it's generally considered to be safe, you should be under the supervision of a medical professional before choosing to fast for longer than one day at a time. Patients with certain conditions like diabetes, hypoglycemia, or those who may be pregnant should not practice fasting. See the Appendix for the fasting protocol.

Yeast, the Hidden Culprit

The typical American diet of refined carbohydrates like pasta, breads and pastry, as well as a heavy sugar intake, gives rise to dismal digestive health. Moreover, with the use of steroids, antibiotics, and NSAID medications, the digestive system is further weakened by decreased gut-immunity and increased fungal or yeast organisms. This condition is called dysbiosis. While yeast is natural to the human body, when its population becomes excessive it may lead to fungal or yeast infections.

For some people, the immune system's reaction to dysbiosis may be experienced as inflammation, joint or muscle pain, sinus congestion and mucus discharge, skin rash, or itching, to name a few of the symptoms.

Many patients have benefited by cutting yeast products from their diet. To start, eliminate yeast-containing products like breads, pasta, pastry, beer, wine, cheese, milk, pickles, vinegar and products made with it, dried fruits, mushrooms, and all sugars and sweeteners. Eat only cooked whole grains, vegetables, nuts and seeds, herbs and spices, and fish and poultry. Take high quality probiotic supplements containing acidophilus, bifudus and other beneficial bacterial strains to help restore your gut flora and correct dysbiosis. See the Appendix for the Yeast-Free Diet.

Go With Goat but Not With Cow

Many parents have observed that when they removed cow's milk and related products from their children's diets, many chronic conditions like sinus problems, recurrent ear infections, and eczema cleared up easily. When they put these items back into their children's diets, their conditions would flare. And yet when their children eat goat or sheep's milk and cheese, similar problems don't arise. The difference may lie with the protein. The protein in cow's milk is large and often not recognized by your immune system, and so your body considers it to be foreign. People with sensitive immune systems will react adversely to the foreign proteins, causing allergic reactions and in severe cases, violent inflammation. Another problem with cow's milk may be lactose, as many people have lactose intolerance. Goat and sheep's milk, however, have protein almost the exact same size as mother's milk, which is why in ancient times when mothers ran out of breast milk, goat milk was the substitute of choice, rather than cow's milk. If you suffer from arthritis, try skipping cow's milk, cheese and ice cream for a month and see how you feel. Chances are, you'll notice an improvement in as little as one week.

Chapter Three:
Healing Herbs and
Supplements

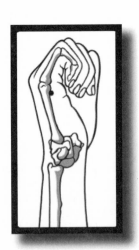

Arthritis is not a new condition. Since time immemorial, humans have struggled to cope with pain in their bodies, and searched for ways to find relief. As a result, there is a large body of knowledge and empirical evidence, including folk cures, that have been passed down over time in many cultures. In China, the results from 5,000 years of meticulous clinical observation and recording of the use of herbal therapy for arthritis has benefited populations beyond its own, including most of Asia and parts of Africa, Europe, and the Middle East. While there are simple herbal remedies involving single herbs like turmeric or ginger, a mainstay of Chinese herbal therapy is the synergistic combination of a number of herbs blended together in formulas for maximum beneficial outcome. Therefore, the best way to use Chinese herbal therapy is to either consult a licensed practitioner of Chinese medicine for a customized herbal blend or to look for patent formulas that are designed for arthritis healing.

In modern times, much research has been devoted to studying natural compounds from foods and herbs that have therapeutic and healing properties. These dietary supplements, or nutriceuticals as they are sometimes called, are another natural way to enhance your body's structure and function. Examples include chondroitin sulfate from shellfish, which is a building block of cartilage; eicosapentaenoic acid (EPA) and docosahexaenoic acid (DHA), omega-3 fatty acids from fish oils that reduce inflammation and prevent plaque buildup in the arteries; and salicin, an active ingredient in white willow bark that has natural analgesic and anti-inflammatory properties. Similar to herbal therapy, an effective nutrition supplement program should be customized after consultations with a qualified practitioner.

Most herbs and supplements are readily available in health food stores, offices of complementary medicine practitioners and online. Purity of ingredients and high bioavailability of the nutrients are important considerations when using herbs and supplements. See the Resources section for a list of recommended products.

Strengthen Tendons and Ligaments with Eucommia Bark

Eucommia, or *Du zhong*, is sometimes known as the Chinese rubber tree. The bark from this tree has the distinct appearance of sections held together by strands of fiber, similar to the way bones are held together by tendons and ligaments. It is traditionally used in Chinese medicine to strengthen the back, hips, knees, and ankles. Eucommia is thought to give strength and flexibility to tendons and ligaments and is popular with athletes. It is also used as a tonic herb to strengthen sexual vitality. Research has also confirmed its ability to regulate blood pressure, and in China it is often prescribed for hypertension. It can be taken in tea or capsule form but is often used as part of a formula with other herbs, such as in the *Arthritis/ Joint* and *DuraBone* formulas. See the Resources section for more information.

Cinnamon for Cold Bi Arthritis

Cinnamon has been a staple of Chinese herbal medicine for thousands of years. It comes from the cassia tree, an evergreen native to Southeast Asia. Cinnamon has a myriad of uses in herbal medicine. Generally, it is used as a warming agent to treat all sorts of cold issues, from the common cold to arthritic pain (of the Cold Bi type) that is worsened by cold weather. Cinnamon is also an energizing herb used to treat fatigue and low energy. More recent research suggests that cinnamon can help reduce insulin resistance in the body and aid insulin's effectiveness, which is quite significant for diabetics. Cinnamon is available in rolled bark sticks, powder, tinctures, and chopped twigs. It can be taken in tea or capsule form, but is often used as part of a formula with other herbs, such as the *Arthritis/Joint* formula. See the Resources section for more information.

Ox Knee is Good for Your Knees

Achyranthes root, or *Niu Xi*, is also known as ox knee, as its shape resembles that of the oxen joint. Long used in Chinese medicine for its joint health-restoring properties, it is notably used as the herb of choice for problems of the knee, including arthritis pain and weakness. Achyranthes is also used to activate blood flow, reduce blockages, and relieve pain. Similar to Eucommia, it has been studied and recommended for its ability to regulate blood pressure. It can be taken in tea or capsule form, but is often used as part of a formula with other herbs, as in the *Arthritis/Joint* formula. See the Resources section for more information.

Mulberry is Very Good for Your Back

Loranthus, or *Sang Ji Sheng*, comes from the showy mistletoe family that lives and grows on other trees. In China they grow specifically on mulberry trees. It is traditionally used in Chinese medicine pain relief from Wind Bi and Damp Bi arthritis. Also known as a tonic for the kidney and liver systems, Loranthus is said to strengthen the back and nourish blood. It can be taken in tea or capsule form but is often used as part of a formula with other herbs such as the *Arthritis/ Joint* and *DuraBone* formulas. See the Resources section for more information.

Angelica for More Than Arthritis Relief

Angelica Pubescens, or *Du Huo,* is part of a plant family that grows mostly in the Northern Hemisphere. Traditionally used in Chinese medicine to treat arthritis, headaches and muscle pain, Angelica has been found in modern research to contain anti-inflammatory and anti-clotting compounds. One such compound, osthole, seems to have additional benefits, such as enhancing vascular dilation, increasing circulation, and possibly enhancing libido. It can be taken in tea or capsule form, but is often paired with Loranthus in a 1,200 year-old Chinese herbal formulation for arthritis called *Du Huo Ji Sheng Tang,* which is the basis for both the *Arthritis/Joint* formula and the *Pain* formula. See the Resources section for more information.

Traditional Pain Relief with Corydalis

Corydalis root, or *Yan Hu Suo,* is part of the fumewort family, and can also be included in the poppy family. It is traditionally used to activate blood flow, remove stagnant blood, and relieve pain. Often used as a safe and natural painkiller and calming agent in Chinese medicine, Corydalis has been found to possess compounds similar to those found in Western anti-inflammatory, analgesic, and allergy mediations, and has also been known to improve heart function and aid in restful sleep. Corydalis can be taken in tea or capsule form by itself for pain relief, but it is often used as part of a formula with other herbs, such as in the *Arthritis/Joint* formula. See the Resources section for more information.

Anti-Aging Siberian Ginseng

Eleuthero root, or *Ci Wu Jia*, is also commonly known as Siberian ginseng. Traditionally known as a tonic for aging and its related symptoms, notably lower back pain and joint weakness, it is also known famously as an herbal tonic liqueur. Research in Russia and Korea has yielded troves of information on the herb. It has been found to be an adaptogen that is helpful in assisting the body to combat stress and recover from adrenal fatigue. Additionally, eleuthero has been found to contain compounds that function as antioxidants and anti-inflammatories, and that help to lower cholesterol and enhance immune system repair. It may also prove helpful in increasing endurance, and improving learning and memory functions. It can be taken in tea or capsule form, but is often used as part of a formula with other herbs, such as the *DuraBone* formula. See the Resources section for more information.

Strong Bones with Bone Mender

Drynaria, or *Gu Sui Bu,* is part of a fern species that's also known as "bone mender." Its name reflects the plant's main function, which is to strengthen and heal broken bones, teeth and connective tissues. Drynaria is primarily used for its ability to heal sprains, bruises, stress fractures, weak loins, and knees. It is also used as a tonic for recuperation from other injuries. Drynaria is used in treatments for tooth-related maladies, such as toothache and bleeding gums, as well as for tinnitus of the ears. Its focus on the kidney and liver channels inspires Chinese medical use in strengthening the kidneys, curbing diarrhea, and promoting tissue regeneration. When used topically, it is said to stimulate hair growth. It can be taken in tea or capsule form, but is often used as part of a formula with other herbs, such as the *DuraBone* formula. See the Resources section for more information.

Healing Traumatic Injuries with Dipsacus

The name for dipsacus root in Chinese, *Xu Duan*, translates to "restore what is broken." Indeed, this herb's primary function is to assist in healing traumatic injuries, especially to the lower parts of your body. According to Chinese medicine, dipsacus root strengthens bones and connective tissue like tendons and ligaments. To this point, it treats conditions like weak, sore, stiff, and painful lower back and knees, as well as osteopenia and osteoporosis. In addition to strengthening the body, dipsacus root can also strengthen the mind by helping to treat memory loss. It can be taken in tea or capsule form, but is often used as part of a formula with other herbs, such as the *DuraBone* formula. See the Resources section for more information.

Chase Away Body and Joint Ache with Notopterygium

Notopterygium, or *Qiang Huo*, is a plant native to east Asia and a relative of the angelica species. It has long been used to treat the flu and its accompanying body aches, fever, and headaches, it is often taken in the initial stages of the flu, when symptoms first begin to present. In traditional Chinese medicine it is very commonly used to treat joint pain, especially pain in the upper limbs, neck, and back, as well as headache pain in the back of the head. It can be taken in tea or capsule form, but is often used as part of a formula with other herbs, such as the *Arthritis/Joint* formula. See the Resources section for more information.

Relax Muscles with Siler Root

The Chinese name for siler, *Fang Feng*, translates to "guard against wind." It is also known as ledebouriella root. Siler root can be used to treat cold-related headaches and body aches, especially pains in the joints, as well as diarrhea, chills, and tremors. It is also a remedy for tetanus, lockjaw, and general convulsions, and additionally helps to relax muscles. Siler root has an antimicrobial effect and has been shown to inhibit influenza viruses. It has been used in China as an antidote to arsenic poisoning. It can be taken in tea or capsule form, but is often used as part of a formula with other herbs, such as the *Arthritis/Joint* formula. See the Resources section for more information.

Activate Immune Repair with Astragalus Root

Astragalus, or *Huang Qi*, is a well-known tonic herb in Chinese medicine that promotes a healthy immune system and strengthens your body against disease. Sometimes called milk vetch, it is used in arthritis conditions to promote repair and regeneration of joints. In addition to its reputation as a whole-body protector, astragalus improves digestion and metabolism. It is used for cases where fatigue, lack of appetite, and diarrhea are present. Studies show that it seems to be particularly useful for those who suffer from frequent colds and flu. Astragalus is an adaptogen that helps the body to maintain normal functions and repair itself during stressful times, to boost energy, support red and white blood cell regeneration, and help reduce side effects from chemotherapy and radiation. It can be taken in tea or capsule form, but is often used as part of a formula with other herbs, such as the *Arthritis/Joint* formula. See the Resources section for more information.

Chinese Foxglove Found Useful for RA

Rehmannia, or *Sheng Di,* resembles the digitalis plant and is commonly referred to as Chinese foxglove. This herb is one of the more famous herbs in Chinese herbology. It is used for a wide variety of complaints. Some of its major uses are for the treatment of both high and low grade fever, thirst, dry mouth and throat, and constipation with dry stools. It can also be used for cases of irritability and insomnia where symptoms of dryness are also present. Preparations of rehmannia have been tested clinically and shown to treat rheumatoid arthritis and eczema when taken internally. It can be taken in tea or capsule form, but is often used as part of a formula with other herbs, such as the *Arthritis/Joint* and *DuraBone* formulas. See the Resources section for more information.

Medieval Herb From Liguria Relieves Pain

Chinese lovage, or *Gao Ben,* also goes by the name ligusticum. The name "lovage" literally meant "love-ache" during medieval times. Ligusticum was extensively cultivated in "Liguria." The name suggests that it was known for its pain relieving properties. The root of Chinese lovage is traditionally used in herbal medicine to reduce pain, especially headaches. Additionally, it is often used in Chinese medicine to treat stomach disorders and feverish attacks. It can be taken in tea or capsule form, but is often used as part of a formula with other herbs, such as the *Arthritis/Joint* formula and the *Pain* formula. See the Resources section for more information.

Chinese Peony Does More Than Look Pretty

Peony, or *Shao Yao*, is a flowering shrub native to China and East Asia. Peony is used as an ornamental plant, and is revered for its large silky flowers and lovely appearance, but peony also serves numerous medicinal functions. The extract of the plant is antibacterial and has been shown to inhibit the growth of E. coli, typhoid, and other bacteria. Therefore it is particularly important in infectious arthritis when the inflammation of muscles and joints is due to bacterial infection. It is used to treat nosebleeds associated with colds, respiratory infections, and sinusitis. When prepared as a tea, peony is used as a cough remedy. When used in response to conditions of the liver, peony is used to support detoxifying functions. It also works as an antioxidant, and helps to modulate your immune system, protect your heart, and calm your nervous system. It can be taken in tea or capsule form, but is often used as part of a formula with other herbs, such as the *Arthritis/Joint, Pain,* and *Muscle Strength* formulas. See the Resources section for more information.

Dong Quai is a Tonic for Both Women and Joints

Dong quai is from the Angelica plant family, and is also known as the female ginseng. It is indigenous to China and the eastern regions of Asia, and is said to be one of the few good non-animal sources of vitamin B12. Studies show Dong quai to possess analgesic, anti-inflammatory and antispasmodic properties, and it has been used extensively in formulas to support arthritis relief. Although Dong quai's use in traditional Chinese medicine has focused on its ability to treat gynecological disorders for thousands of years, its qualities as a uterine and blood tonic, and also as a hormonal regulator, illustrate its use in helping with the female reproductive system. Dong quai has also been found to inhibit the growth of various bacteria, including Bacillus dysenteriae and Bacillus typhi. It can be taken in tea or capsule form, but is often used as part of a formula with other herbs, such as the *Arthritis/Joint*, *Pain*, and *DuraBone* formulas. See the Resources section for more information.

Improve Circulation with Myrrh

Myrrh is the dried sap or resin of the Commiphora myrrha tree, and is native to Eastern Africa and the southern region of the Middle East. It is a bitter substance that, along with its medicinal properties, is used in incense, perfumes, and as an additive to wine. It enjoyed cultural prominence and was valued by the ancient Greek and Roman civilizations. Myrrh has similar uses to that of frankincense, though according to traditional Chinese medicine, myrrh moves blood while frankincense moves energy. Similarly, in Ayurvedic medicine, myrrh is used for circulatory problems. Myrrh is used for toothache pain, arthritis, tendonitis, sciatica, rheumatism, herpes, asthma, cough, bronchial conditions, cold hands and feet, and gum disease. It is also used to balance the immune system. It can be taken in tea or capsule form, but is often used as part of a formula with other herbs, such as the *Arthritis/Joint* formula and the *DuraBone* formula. See the Resources section for additional information.

Frankincense - Biblical Cure for Arthritis

Boswellia has several names. It is also known as frankincense, oliba-num, or *Ru Xiang*, in Chinese. It is the aromatic resin that is obtained from the Boswellia genus of trees. The name "frankincense" derives from its introduction to Europe by Frankish crusaders. Originally from the Middle East, Boswellia has historically been used in religious rites described in the Old Testament. In Chinese medicine, it has been used for arthritic inflammation, pain relief, and to improve circulation. Commercially, Frankincense has increasingly been used in perfumes, incense, and pastilles. Frankincense is also popular for its use in aromatherapy. Food-grade frankincense must be translucent in color, meaning that no black or brown impurities are present. In fact, *Ru Xiang* means "fragrant milk," which alludes to its purity in color.

Frankincense can be found as a resin, powder, or essential oil, and can be taken orally in capsule form, but is often used as part of a formula with other herbs, such as the *Pain* formula and the *Channel Opener* formula. See the Resources section for more information.

Make Your Integuments Strong with Vitamins A and Carotenes

A critical vitamin for the growth and repair of body tissues, vitamin A supports healthy mucus membranes, maintains youthful skin, and promotes collagen production. It is also important to the optimum functioning of your immune system. In arthritis, it blocks an inflammatory compound when there is adequate amount of vitamin A present in the body. Most of the time, it is better to get vitamin A through its precursor, known as carotenes, which can be found in yellow, orange, and green vegetables, such as carrots, apricot, spinach, pumpkins, squash, sweet potato, and kale.

Essential B Vitamins for Healing Arthritis

Many of the B vitamins are essential for healing arthritis. They function best together as a team, and when properly balanced in a complex form, they can enhance the benefits and reduce the negatives. One of the key functions of B vitamins is to help enzymes release energy from food. Their other functions include maintaining a healthy metabolism and nervous system, and keeping your skin, hair, eyes, and digestive tract healthy as well.

For example, B1 is good for circulation and its deficiency can lead to swelling. B2 is needed for digestion of protein, fats, and carbohydrates. B3 maintains the health of blood vessels and reduces fatty and cholesterol deposits on the arteries and in the liver. It also lowers blood pressure. B5 improves the body's resistance to stress, and is therefore often called the anti-stress vitamin. B6 is necessary for protein metabolism and is known for its ability to reduce the symptoms of premenstrual syndrome (PMS), such as bloating and water retention. Biotin (B7) is important in maintaining good skin, hair, and nails and, correspondingly, joints. Folic Acid (B9) is critical for growth and reproduction, and therefore is essential in pregnancy to prevent birth defects. Finally, B12 helps create new red blood cells and promotes energy and a healthy nervous system.

Antioxidant Vitamin C for Tissue Repair

A Scottish navel surgeon who linked nutrients found in citrus fruits to the prevention of scurvy was credited as the first to discover Vitamin C, or ascorbic acid. That nutrient would later become one of the most studied vitamins. Vitamin C is everywhere in the body and is involved in a multitude of functions. It is a potent antioxidant, helps to protect the brain and spinal cord from damage, and assists in the fight against infections and toxins. It is also essential in collagen production and connective tissue repair, therefore performs a critical part in the healing of arthritis. Foods rich in ascorbic acid include broccoli, cauliflower, pepper, parsley, and citrus, and you can also take it in a supplement form.

Vitamin D Lowers the Risk of Developing RA

Your body creates vitamin D from exposure to the sun. Healthy levels of vitamin D are essential for maintaining healthy bones and cartilage, so it may be no surprise that people living closer to the equator, where they spend more time in the sun every day, have fewer incidents of arthritis than their northern brethren. However, if you live in the Northern states or get little to no sun, do not despair, as you can easily obtain vitamin D from food or supplements. New research suggests that vitamin D may offer some protection against rheumatoid arthritis (RA), after a large study of women showed that vitamin D obtained from food and supplements appears to lower the risk of developing RA. In fact, women who had a high intake of the vitamin were found to be less likely to develop the disease.

Oxygenate Your Tissues and Organs with Vitamin E

Vitamin E is a potent antioxidant and has been found to be helpful in preventing cancer and heart disease. Specifically, it facilitates the distribution of oxygen to the organs and protects tissues from environmental toxins. It is also beneficial for fertility and reproduction. When used topically, vitamin E hastens the healing process of the skin, and when ingested, it prevents blood clots. Its ability to strengthen blood vessels and aid in the oxygenation of tissues makes it an important nutrient for cartilage repair and regeneration. Foods rich in vitamin E include olives, chard, mustard greens, sunflower seeds, and almonds.

Lower Your Body's Inflammation with Vitamin K

Deficiency in this vitamin is rare, but overuse of antibiotics can adversely affect intestinal health, which is where we naturally produce this vitamin. Vitamin K has been shown to reduce many inflammatory markers in the blood. It's found in large amounts in avocados and in soybean oil, and may serve to explain the anti-inflammatory effects of a nutritional compound called Avocado and Soybean Unsaponifiables (ASU). Vitamin K has also been shown to benefit bone mass. It is found in foods like leafy green vegetables, avocado, kiwi, meat, dairy, and eggs.

ASU Increases the Building Blocks of Cartilage

ASU (Avocado and Soybean Unsaponifiables) is an extract made from the oils in avocados and soybeans and has been shown to reduce inflammatory substances in the body. Its use has been shown to reduce the need for pain medications in osteoarthritis (OA) patients, and ASU supplements have been prescribed by doctors in Europe for years. Exactly what are ASUs? They are aggrecan molecules that are abundant in the human body and which form the structural building blocks of cartilage. Specifically, an aggrecan molecule consists of hundreds of chains of cartilage-building nutrients like chondroitin sulfate. Therefore, maintaining high levels of aggrecans are essential for healthy joints. Research from Europe has shown that oils from avocado and soy greatly boosted production of aggrecans, which thereby increased the repair of damage caused by OA. ASU comes in capsule form, but you can always increase your consumption of avocado and soybeans instead.

Support Your Joint Health with Glucosamine & Chondroitin

Commercial production of glucosamine is largely sourced from crustacean shells. High-quality products should be free of the shellfish protein that may cause allergic reactions in those susceptible, but if there's any question, you should consult your primary physician before you start taking it.

Occurring naturally in our cartilage, chondroitin gives the tissue its strong resistance to compression. As a supplement, it comes primarily from bovine sources of cartilage. When glucosamine and chondroitin are taken together, studies have shown them to benefit cartilage restoration, thereby reducing pain and improving joint function However, their use can take several months to show measurable change on x-rays of cartilage. Another challenge is that the majority of people who will choose to take Glucosamine are usually over the age of 50, and as you get older, the hydrochloric acid production in the stomach declines, which can potentially cause poor breakdown and absorption of glucosamine. Recent studies have been done on the use of glucosamine sulfate versus glucosamine hydrochloride, and glucosamine HCL has been shown to be more effective than the original sulfate forms. One way to overcome this is to take separate hydrochloride supplements together with a glucosamine sulfate supplement.

Lubricate Joints with Hyaluronic Acid

Hyaluronic acid is a major lubricating component of the synovial fluid secreted within the joint capsule. It coats the outside of each cartilage cell, otherwise known as the chondrocyte, and along with other synovial components, is responsible for the chondrocytes' ability to retain water, giving the cartilage its ability to withstand pressure. Outside the joint, it helps in tissue repair and is thought to aid in development of the brain. You can obtain hyaluronic acid naturally in food by eating chicken wings, sardines with bones, and beef tendons. Be sure to eat the cartilage from the ends of the bones. You can also make a broth from beef bones and cartilage. It is also available as a supplement from health food stores or online.

All-Around Relief with MSM

Methylsulfonylmethane (MSM) has gained considerable recognition for its results in relieving arthritis. MSM is a natural form of organic sulfur found in all living organisms, and is present in low concentrations in our body fluids and tissues. It has been found to reduce inflammation and relieve pain. It also dilates blood vessels, therefore sending a great supply of blood into your joints, and helping to relax muscle spasms. MSM is found in a variety of fresh foods, including fruits, vegetables, meat, fish, and milk. However, unless your diet is composed primarily of raw foods, it is unlikely that you are receiving enough MSM for proper health management. MSM is available orally, as capsules or crystals, and can also applied topically to the skin as a lotion, cream, or gel.

Fish Oil Extinguishes Inflammatory Fire

Fish oil contains omega-3 fatty acids that offer significant benefits to patients suffering from inflammatory and autoimmune diseases and depression. Many of the placebo-controlled trials of fish oil in studies related to chronic inflammatory diseases revealed significant benefits, including decreased disease activity and a lowered use of anti-inflammatory drugs. The fatty acids that are specific to fish oil and not flax oil, are eicosapentaenoic acid (EPA) and docosahexaenoic acid (DHA). These are effective in decreasing the pro-inflammatory chemical interleuki 1 (IL-1), which is not only involved in arthritis but also in heart disease, multiple sclerosis and Crohn's disease. EPA and DHA also stimulate blood circulation, help to breakdown fibrin, a component of scar tissue, and can also lower blood pressure. Its use has also shown synergistic effects when paired with Glucosamine. Rheumatoid arthritis patients have been shown to benefit from a daily supplement of EPA and DHA.

GLA to the Rescue

GLA, or Gamma Linolinic Acid, is an important fatty acid that has been found to reduce inflammation and help combat rheumatoid arthritis, nerve damage, and Alzheimer's-induced memory loss. In fact, several clinical studies have demonstrated the effectiveness of GLA on the symptoms of rheumatoid arthritis. They have also shown its use to cause a reduction in the use of non-steroidal anti-inflammatory drugs. Natural sources high in GLA include evening primrose oil, borage, and black current seed oil. These oils can be used in salads but not as cooking oils, because heat degrades their quality. GLA also comes in liquid or capsule form.

SAMe as Celebrex in Studies

SAMe, or S-adenosylmethionine, is a sulfur-containing compound. In a double-blind study comparing SAMe to the prescription anti-inflammatory drug Celebrex, the results showed no difference between the two groups; meaning that SAMe was as effective as the drug, but without the harmful side effects. SAMe seems to work as well as over-the-counter and other prescription drugs for osteoarthritis, but it works more slowly. The mechanism for its anti-inflammatory property is the ability to reduce the body's production of a substance that's involved in cartilage destruction. It also has been found to increase cartilage production. Widely used in Europe, it is available in supplement form from health food stores and online.

Glutamine is Good for Joints and Nerves

One of the most abundant amino acids found in the muscles, glutamine helps to build and maintain muscle mass and prevent muscle atrophy. It is converted in the brain to glutamic acid, which has been shown to be important to healthy brain functioning. Glutamine has antioxidant properties and can help counter nerve damage, such as peripheral neuropathy and brain fog, often found in cancer patients undergoing chemotherapy and radiation. It has been found to be beneficial in the fight against arthritis and other autoimmune diseases. Good natural sources of glutamine include cabbage, beets, fish, and beans. You can also take it in a supplement form.

Healthy Elastin with Lysine

Elastin is another type of connective tissue protein, and is most notable for its ability to retract to its original shape. The ears and nose are a good example of this. The essential amino acid (meaning humans do not inherently produce it and must consume it from outside sources) responsible for the durability of elastin is Lysine. This amino acid is necessary for the body to build proteins. The cartilage and surrounding muscles of our joins are largely protein and fluids. Lysine-rich foods include beans, meat, eggs, and fish, such as cod and sardines. It is readily available as a supplement in health food stores or online.

Twin Aminos for Your Joints and Nails

Cysteine and Cystine are amino acids that are closely related and capable of converting into one another when the need arises. They are powerful antioxidants that deactivate free radicals, expel toxins, and help your body to create more proteins. Both contain sulfur, which helps reduce inflammation, as well as assisting in the production of collagen and the protein in nails, skin, and hair. Rich natural supplies of cysteine and cystine are found in garlic, brussels sprouts, wheat germ, and egg yolk. You can also take them in supplement form.

Trace Boron for Healthy Bones and Joints

Boron is a trace mineral essential for healthy bones, muscles, and joints. It works with calcium, magnesium, and vitamin D to promote bone health. Boron also promotes sharper brain function and increases focus and memory. Studies also suggest that boron is helpful in lessening arthritis joint pain. Almonds, apricot, avocado, dates, and Brazil nuts are rich in boron. It can also be taken in supplement form, usually combined with other vitamins in a formula.

Adequate Calcium for Structural Support

Calcium is probably the most important and common mineral that we need to keep our bodies functioning properly. It is essential in the building of strong bones and joints. Most people are familiar with its structural function; however, calcium is also critical for the transmission of nerve signals and helps to maintain healthy muscle tissue, a shortage of which can cause muscle cramping. Diets high in fat, protein, and sugar reduces calcium absorption from food. Natural foods rich in calcium include leafy greens, dried beans, legumes, egg shells, and almonds. When taking calcium supplements, be sure to balance your intake with magnesium for maximum absorption of calcium.

Increase Energy with Magnesium

Magnesium is necessary for energy production within each cell in your body. It helps with the absorption of calcium, potassium and other minerals. Magnesium maintains healthy nerve and muscle function. It is also used to soften stool, calm blood pressure, and alleviate anxiety. Rich natural sources of magnesium include black beans, halibut, spinach, and pumpkin seeds. Always include magnesium with calcium supplements for maximum absorption.

Copper for Your Immune System and Joint Health

Copper is a trace mineral, and is essential for building bones, making elastin, and producing red blood cells. It is necessary for the production of collagen in your skin, joints, and muscles. A natural antibacterial agent, copper is also beneficial in the immune system's fight against infections. As a result of its properties, copper helps to increase the quality of your hair and skin, keep your appearance youthful, and bring relief to your arthritis pain. Foods high in copper include sesame seeds, sunflower seeds, tomatoes, pumpkin seeds, and coca. It is usually included as part of a supplement formulation and not taken individually unless directed by your healthcare provider.

Powerful Enzymes to Reduce Inflammation

Your spleen and pancreas, together with the stomach and liver, produce a wide array of enzymes, each specifically used to break down and access various foods and nutrients. There are many enzymes at work, but the main ones include the digestion of fats with lipase, protein with protease, and starch with carbohydrase. Additionally, there is papain and bromalain, both of which are helpful in reducing inflammation in the body, particularly in the joints. You can opt to eat fresh fruits and vegetables, many of which contain natural digestive enzymes to help you reduce inflammatory response, or you can take them in supplement form. See the Resources section for more information.

A Note on Over-the-Counter Drugs

Pharmaceutical medications are used by millions of people to allay the painful effects of arthritis. Because they work so well over the short term for relief from pain and inflammation, people often try to tolerate the devastating side effects their use can lead to in the long run. Common side effects include harmful interactions with many other drugs, perforation of the gut, damage to the liver or kidney, high blood pressure, and ulcers. The most common drugs used are NSAIDS (non-steroidal anti-inflammatory drugs) like aspirin, ibuprofen (Motrin, Advil, etc.), naproxen (Aleve, Midol, etc.), diclofenac, ketoprofen, and tiaprofenic acid. These are prescribed by the tens of millions every year, accounting for over 100,000 hospital visits due to their side effects and killing 16,500 people annually in the U.S.

Second in popularity to NSAIDS is acetaminophen (Tylenol), found commonly in hundreds of over-the-counter products. Acetaminophen may be cheaper or have a shorter list of side effects (when taken at a low dose) than NSAIDS, but it's largely ineffective for arthritic pain relief and may even make the pain worse. Still, the FDA found that acetaminophen accounts for 26,000 annual hospital visits and 450 deaths per year in the U.S. But more to the point, these drugs do absolutely nothing for the underlying cause of arthritis. Prescription drugs, including anti-inflammatory compounds such as Celebrex, steroids like prednisone and immunosuppressants such as methotrexate must be closely monitored for their side effects.

Chapter Four:
Joint Care, Acupressure and Acupuncture

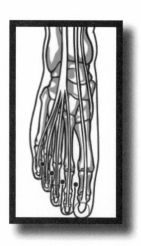

Do you spend an hour or more each day watching television? Try doing some simple stretches instead, or even while watching your favorite shows. Have you injured yourself during a yoga or aerobics class? Get proper coaching in your favorite activities to avoid hurting yourself or to rebuild after an injury. Do you sit for long periods at a desk or in your car? Take a two-minute walk several times during your workday or after a lengthy commute. If questions like these go unanswered you may be taking much from your joints without putting energy back into them. You can view your joint use like a checking account. There is only so much money to withdraw before problems arise. Given a choice, most people would happily avoid bouncing a check or experiencing pain in the joints they rely on every day. In that way, decisions such as choosing to eat the right foods and supplements, losing excessive weight, and committing to joint building exercises are all like making deposits into the checking account of your joint health.

Strengthen, Mobilize, and Activate

There are many different types of exercise for you to choose from that are easy on your joints, including walking, tai chi, and yoga. Some can be done entirely on your own, while others, such as pilates, spinning, or gyrotonics, may require equipment or instruction. You may even choose one of the many recommended activities mentioned in this chapter, depending on the severity of your arthritic limitations and personal interest. If your interest lies in Tai Chi or Qi Gong, we recommend taking a class at your acupuncturist's office or community recreation center. Many studies have shown that forms of movement exercise such as Tai Chi and Qi Gong to be beneficial for arthritis. These are slow, choreographed movements combined with breathing and relaxed focus, almost like a type of moving meditation. In this chapter, we will show you several effective foundational practices for Tai Chi and Qi Gong that can get your energy and blood circulation flowing in a short period of time.

When it comes to self-healing, there is no more powerful or effective system than acupressure. Acupressure employs the same principles as acupuncture, only without the needles. In this chapter, you will learn how to stimulate acupoints in your body. Each point activates a particular bodily function or neurochemical response, and is done with the brief press of a finger.

Running Water Never Grows Stale

Some people are wary of exercising when experiencing joint pain because they feel it will worsen their problem. While movements need to be performed correctly to avoid additional discomfort, the idea that exercise will worsen arthritic pain is a huge misconception. In fact, a lack of regular movement can make the condition worse. The cartilage receives its nutrients from outside the joint capsule by way of synovial fluid exchange that comes from exercising. Without enough exercise, degrading cartilage won't be given any messages from the body to change its destructive course, and it will continue to wear away. As well, support tissues to the joint will atrophy or shrink when not used regularly. This explains why many people with joint pain experience stiffness when they wake up in the morning after a night of inactivity during sleep. So move your body like running water! Your joints will thank you for it.

Bear Weight, Move Free

There are hundreds of joints in the human body. They come in several forms, but those most susceptible to arthritis are the kinds of joints that bear weight and move freely. These are called synovial joints. The hip and knee are the foremost examples. They're the largest joints in the body, they take on the most weight, and they offer a wide range of movement. On the opposite end of the joint spectrum would be the fixed joints, the best example of which is the joined plates of bone that make up the skull. There is almost no movement and very little weight is placed on them. However, as a newborn, these plates in the skull do shift, to allow the baby's head to pass through the birth canal. The simple fact is that our bodies are born and bred to move. Movement keeps the blood flowing, the oxygen moving, and the healing happening.

If your pain is severe you may need to modify the way you play your sport, or possibly seek out different forms of exercise to support your current condition. Remember to explore your body and your world. There are always more ways to stay active, and you may just find joy in a new activity you didn't think much about before. Talk to a friend, your doctor, or take a movement class at your local gym or community recreation center.

Pump up Your Endorphins with Exercise

Exercise has been shown over and over to improve joint function for arthritis sufferers. With time, pain is reduced and flexibility restored. Exercise also helps us to keep a positive attitude, thanks to a steady stream of endorphins. Otherwise known as the "happy hormones," these act as potent pain-relievers when released from the brain during exercise. Without these hormones and without a regular regimen of movement, depression can easily set in, which only makes it easier to avoid these helpful activities, creating a downward spiral of physical and mental inactivity. Exercise is crucial for your mind, for your joints, for your immune system, for your weight management, for your cartilage, and for a long, happy life.

But how do you get started if you are already depressed or in a great deal of pain? Begin by choosing activities that make this process fun. Read a book while on the stationary bike, go for a nice hike among beautiful scenery, or take a Tai Chi or yoga class. You can even go walking with a group of friends in the mall if it's too cold outside. Enjoying yourself when you exercise is the only way to ensure you keep with a new regimen. A habit that you hate will be harder to stick to in the long run. Start slowly and gradually if you're already in a lot of pain. Choose low-impact exercises like water aerobics or elliptical trainers, lower repetitions when doing stretches or weights, or just 10 minutes of cardiovascular exercise to begin with. If you need more exercise ideas or instruction on being safe during your physical activity, please consult your healing team and a qualified trainer.

Protect Your Joints with Appropriate Activities

Nutrients from the blood vessels surrounding the cartilage reach the innermost cartilage cells by diffusion. This is accomplished by a combination of flexion, extension, and compression when we move our bodies. Gentle, circular, or wave-like movements do this most effectively with least wear to the cartilage. Repetitive, quick, jarring activities can shorten the life of the tissues. Choosing appropriate activities will lengthen the life of our cartilage and ensure that the rest of our body reaps the benefits of a pain-free and mobile lifestyle. Here are some examples of activities that tend to be either constructive or destructive to the life of our cartilage:

Constructive: massage, Tai Chi, Qi Gong, water aerobics, yoga, stretching, walking, hiking, bicycling.

Destructive: running on hard surfaces, prolonged standing, poor posture, manual labor, repetitive activities like typing and computer use, and sports that require abrupt sprints like football, basketball, and volleyball.

Some people whose jobs include manual labor often feel that if their jobs already involve physical work they don't need to exercise on their down time. While it's nice to kill two birds with one stone, unless you are an exercise instructor it's likely that the physical movement you do at work strains your body, rather than benefitting it. It's important to choose the right physical activity, and do it correctly and at the proper pace, in order to derive the best physical benefits from your daily exercise routine. A fast-paced aerobics class with loud music and jarring movements is certainly different then a calm hike. Both of these examples have their place and aren't meant for everyone. The right exercise should fit the right person. Work with your health team to find the exercise that's right for you.

Merry-Go-Round for a Long Life

All centenarians walk. Walking is an easy, low-impact way to get quality cardiovascular exercise, burn fat, keep the joints flexible, and see some of your neighborhood all at the same time. Make sure to walk at a brisk pace and wear comfortable shoes and clothing. All the joints are incorporated into the movement process when you walk. Similarly to practicing Qi Gong and Tai Chi, this coordinated movement along with steady breathing can both exercise the musculoskeletal system and also "massage" all of the internal organs. The heart is primarily responsible for pumping blood and nutrients around the body, but the lungs act like two large hearts as well. As the lungs expand, pressure is placed on all the internal organs, further helping body fluids to move and chemical exchange to take place. This, in turn, is what directly helps push in and pull out the synovial fluid within the joint capsules to keep the joints nourished and healthy.

A simple walking exercise called Merry-Go-Round can be done by anyone in any condition. It involves walking in a steady pace in a circle of any size while holding your arms in different poses. Merry-Go-Round is a foundational practice for a martial art from China called Ba Gua, or Cosmic Tour. It can be done indoors around a dinner table or outdoors around a tree, or in any open space. Be sure the surface is flat without any obstacles that may cause you to trip. You can practice Merry-Go-Round for anywhere from five to 25 minutes anytime of the day.

Watch online: log on to collegeoftao.com

Moving with Grace and Poise with Tai Chi

Tai Chi is practiced by more than 100 million people worldwide, mostly in China, but the number of American practitioners is on the rise. It is a choreographed sequence of circular arm movements and dance-like steps coordinated with a pattern of breathing. When practicing Tai Chi all of the body's joints are exercised and strengthened at the same time. When watching someone practice Tai Chi one cannot help but admire the graceful movements and poise of the practitioner. Many studies have shown that practicing Tai Chi reduces pain, improves joint function, increases mental acuity, and the overall quality of life. In particular, Tai Chi promotes better proprioception, which is the awareness of your body's limbs during movements relative to your physical environment, which prevents falls and injuries. This is important because as people age proprioception decreases, contributing to more falls and bone breakage.

Watch online: log on to collegeoftao.com

Take a Hike for Fresh Air and a Better View

Hiking is a wonderful activity, but one that is better accustomed to those with little-to-no discomfort in their lower extremities, due to the demand hiking places on the hips, knees, ankles, and toes. There are different types of terrain to hike on and there are many guide-books to give you more information, as well as details on altitude, trail length, and skill level. There should be something for every-one, assuming you live in an area with good access to trails. Proper footwear is a must to ensure the feet and lower joints are well cared for. The right equipment will also help to prevent injury or falls on certain terrains. Exercising in a clean environment with fresh air is much preferred over a polluted, urban space. If you live in a city and can't get away to a more pristine location, the best time to exercise outdoors in the city would be between 5 and 7 a.m. when the air is still clean and hasn't yet been disturbed by the morning commute. When the air is filled with pollution during rush hour traffic it's much healthier to exercise indoors.

Pedal Your Way to Health

Bicycling is an excellent exercise to stimulate your cardiovascular system. It's an effective, low-impact way to get your lungs and heart pumping for overall health with minimal strain put on your joints. The seated position removes the upper body's weight from bearing on the lower extremities, allowing a more focused conditioning of the hips, knees, and ankles. On any bike, make sure there is a slight bend in the knee upon full extension of the leg when the foot is on the pedal. As well, when the leg is fully contracted with the foot on the pedal, the thigh and lower leg should not form an angle less than ninety degrees. These positions will keep you from injuring your knee and other joints and tissues. When using a stationary bike, opt for the recumbent position—with a chair to lean against if you suffer from back pain.

Go Easier on Your Joints with an Elliptical Trainer

The elliptical trainer is so named for the elliptical pattern of the foot pedals when in motion. This is a fitness machine that can now be found in virtually every gym and which offers a low-impact alternative to walking or running while also providing an excellent source of cardiovascular exercise for the whole body. Most elliptical machines also work the lower and upper body with moving handlebars. This allows arthritis sufferers to partake in these activities in a way that still protects their joints from experiencing more pain. There are also different ways to get a more intense workout as you get stronger and experience less pain. One way is to increase the resistance setting on the machine. Another is to put weighed vest, wrist, and ankle weights on your body for increased exertion.

Stretch Awake to Start Your Day

For people with arthritis, getting out of bed in the morning can be the most challenging time of the entire day, as stiffness and pain are common early morning experiences. Proper stretching is the best way to bring relief to your symptoms and ensure an active day will follow. Stretching is also easily done on its own as a great way to keep the joints, ligaments, and muscles flexible and engaged. It is also important to stretch before and after any exercises, to allow your body time to warm up and cool down. Working with a physical therapist or trainer whose expertise is in designing a personalized set of stretches is a good way to maximize benefits while avoiding injury.

Extra Tip: using a heating pad, sauna, or hot bath before stretching will improve your ability to elongate your ligaments, tendons, and muscles while reducing strains and sprains. Hot yoga, done inside a heated studio, is an example of this practice. Additionally, use an ice pack or cold shower after exercise to keep the joints or tissues from swelling and becoming inflamed.

Yoga for Health and Healing

Yoga is a discipline, originally from India, that combines stretching, breathing, and meditation practices. There are many different traditions and styles of yoga practice, each with a different focus. Some are gentle movements done slowly, deliberately, and even meditatively, while others are more fast-paced and physically intense workouts. Regardless of the style, Yoga typically involves a sequence of body poses that are held briefly over a period of up to a minute or more to engage the body and mind. It is widely practiced in yoga studios, gyms, and community recreation centers.

A discipline similar to Yoga, but originating in China, is called *Dao-In*. Some poses in Dao-In may be similar to Indian yoga but rather than holding the poses stationary, it encourages gentle, slow movements done alongside careful breathing and focused intent. The goal is to use proper movements to activate acupoints and encourage the flow of energy through the meridians for optimum health and healing.

Learn online: see a demo of Dao-In at collegeoftao.com

Weight Training for Strength

If you are interested in building your strength, free weights are a great way to start weight training. There are also several different types of machines designed to work any specific muscle or group of muscles to support joint strength and function. If you are a beginner and don't have any experience lifting weights, you should start by consulting a certified trainer or physical therapist before you begin in order to avoid injuries. It's generally a good idea to work the whole body during a weight session, rather than targeting one specific area, unless you are working with a professional on an individualized program. Remember not to concentrate too hard on your problem areas; it's important to focus on the whole of your body, rather than just the weak or painful spots. When weight training, it's best not to work the same muscle groups every day. For example, work on the back and legs one day and then focus on the chest and arms the next in order to allow the muscles a day in between workouts to recover properly. Always start with light weights and gradually build up overtime.

Take Weight off Your Joints with Water Exercise

Doing exercise in the water offers opportunities to do aerobics, stretching, or strength training while a portion of the body's weight is taken off the joints thanks to the buoyancy of the water. These movements are usually done in shallow water or with flotation devices, so swimming ability is typically not required. The water allows for easier movement, which can be a benefit for both the body and mind. The increased freedom of movement can help to build self-confidence as people who have been immobilized by disease become encouraged by their ability to move again. If you aren't experienced with water exercise, our suggestion is for you to join a supervised class. Many local programs featuring water-based exercise classes may be available at community recreation centers with a pool, your local YMCA, or other health clubs.

Build a Strong Core with Pilates

Pilates is a fitness system originally developed by Joseph Pilate as a way to rehabilitate soldiers after World War I. Later, it was adapted by the dance community. It uses a combination of breathing practice, mental focus, and strength training by way of stretching and the use of a special apparatus called a reformer. The emphasis of Pilates is on building the core muscles of the abdomen and back in order to support spinal health, proper balance, and overall strength. Whether you are using a Pilates machine in a gym or simpler exercises on a mat, these movements are very accommodating for all fitness levels and for arthritis sufferers. This type of exercise is mostly offered in Pilates studios and health clubs.

Qi Gong for Optimum Wellness

Qi Gong, or qi meditation, is loosely translated as "energy discipline." Rooted in the earliest of Chinese medical healing modalities, Qi Gong allows the participant to combine simple postures, breathing, and mental intention into an exercise regimen that utilizes moments of both movement and stillness. There are many different types of Qi Gong, including those designed for specific conditions, as well as those meant to promote general health and wellbeing. There are also many instructors to choose from. Finding the right style, and the right teacher, can offer those with arthritis a life-changing experience when practiced regularly. Qi Gong is easy to learn and with a minimum number of sequences that can be easily learned by people of any age and physical condition. Like other modalities of Chinese medicine, Qi Gong encourages your body to heal itself through the coordinated inner and outer movements of the mind and body, which is why we sometimes call it a "mind-body" exercise. It is taught by many acupuncturists and certified instructors in community recreation centers and fitness studios.

Watch online: log on to collegeoftao.com

Foundation Exercises from Tai Chi and Qi Gong

When beginning any Tai Chi or Qi Gong practice, it is traditional to start by practicing the foundation exercises. These are used to loosen and open up the various joints of the body, allowing blood, qi, and body fluids to pass through the joints with ease. These exercises are also very useful when beginning any other types of exercise. When practiced regularly, you will experience more graceful movements, minimized joint strain, and increased strength and energy. Moreover, physical and emotional stressors are released during the short routines outlined in the following pages. Start by tapping the trunk, arms, and legs to activate energy and awaken lymphatic circulation. Move on to loosening the joints by circling each joint of the body, then finally bouncing and shaking the body for bone and muscle strengthening. These exercises should be performed with ease and can easily be modified to accommodate weak or painful joints.

Tapping the Trunk to Awaken Energy

Place your feet shoulder width apart with your arms hanging loose at your sides. Shift your weight back and forth from one foot to the other while turning the pelvis at the same time. The weight should be mostly on the left leg while turning the pelvis to the left, and then shifted to the opposite leg as your position changes. This should create momentum enough for your arms to swing in front and behind you. With loose fists, allow them to alternately tap the lower abdomen below the navel and at a similar height on the back. Repeat this movement several times. Continue this turning and tapping while raising the position of where your fists land, moving from the lower abdomen up to the shoulders, tracing a "V" formation, and mirroring this tapping by moving your fists up your back as well. Then tap back down the same path, ending on the lower abdomen and back once again.

Watch online: log on to collegeoftao.com

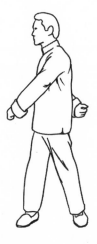

Tapping the Arms

With your feet shoulder width apart, extend your left arm forward at shoulder height. Making a loose fist with your right hand, lightly tap your trunk, starting just beneath the navel, moving along your left side and upward to underneath your left armpit. Move the tapping up your left shoulder to the neck, back down your shoulder and down the inside of your left arm to the palm. Tap up the outside of your left arm, up to the shoulder and neck. When finished, gently shake out your left arm. Repeat this sequence on your right side while tapping with your left fist.

Watch online: log on to collegeoftao.com

Tapping the Back and Legs

Start by rubbing your palms a few times in a circular motion over your lower back and kidney area. The circle should move up the spine, then downwards alongside the spine. With loose fists, tap (using the inner side of your fist with your thumb and first finger) over your lower back in a similar circular pattern several times. Next, place your feet wide apart with your legs straight. Bend at the waist, and using the palm side of your fists, tap down the outer aspect of the buttocks, thighs, legs, and ankles. Tap up the inner ankles, legs, and thighs, straightening your body as you go. Bring your feet back to shoulder width apart. Tap the area that connects the thighs to the pelvis several times and, with each tap, alternate between slightly bent and straightened knees.

Watch online: log on to collegeoftao.com

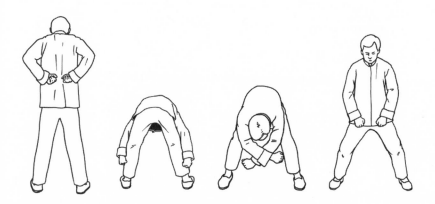

Swing the Arms and Jump for Cardio Stimulation

Place your feet shoulder width apart. Gently swing your arms downward in front of your body and behind to the back, letting the swing take your arms upward. Reverse the swing from the back to the front. Repeat this several times, inhaling as your arms move backward and exhaling as they come forward. Allow a natural resistance to inform you how far to swing them in either direction. Enhance the swing by bending your knees as your arms swing down past the front of your body; and as your arms reach up in the back, lift your heels. After several more swings, jump up as your arms move back and up. You should feel the backward/upward movement of your arms naturally carries you into a jump at the end of the swing. Jump several times, going higher with each swing. Then progressively jump smaller until you stop jumping, slowing the back and forth of the arm swing until you're standing naturally still. This practice has been shown to improve cardiovascular capacity.

Watch online: log on to collegeoftao.com

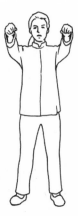
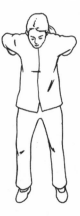

Joint Rotations to Open and Restore Joints

Once vital energy, blood circulation and the lymphatic system are awakened and activated by tapping your trunk and extremities, we need to be sure that the flow isn't obstructed at the joints. Within the foundation practices are movements that circle the joints and open up the flow of synovial fluids to nourish and restore joint functions. These joint rotations should be done gently and slowly without any strain whatsoever. With consistent practice you will naturally experience an increase in the range of motion in your joints.

Watch online: log on to collegeoftao.com

Neck Rotation

Place your heels together and face your feet forward. Place your left hand on the lower abdomen, with the right hand on top of the left. Allowing gravity to do the work in moving your head, gently tilt your torso to the left side, allowing your head to lean to the left, then the back, right, and front. Repeat three times in each direction, inhaling as the head goes back and exhaling as it comes forward again. This is a whole body movement, allowing your head to follow the gravitational pull.

Watch online: log on to collegeoftao.com

Neck Exercise

1. Inhale, moving your head to look upward. Hold your breath and the position for several seconds. Exhale, returning your head to the starting position. Repeat by looking downward.

2. Inhale, turning your head to the right. Hold your breath and the position for several seconds. Exhale, returning your head to the starting position. Repeat by looking in opposite direction.

3. Inhale, tilting your head toward your left shoulder with both shoulders relaxed. Hold your breath and the position for several seconds. Exhale, returning your head to the starting position. Repeat on the other side.

4. Inhale, tilt your head forward and turn to the left, looking downward. Hold your breath and the position for several seconds. Exhale, returning your head to the starting position. Repeat on the other side.

5. Inhale, turn your head to the left and look upward. Hold your breath and the position for several seconds. Exhale, returning your head to the starting position. Repeat on the other side.

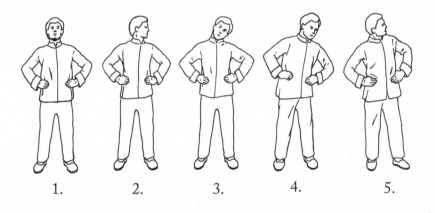

1.   2.   3.   4.   5.

Watch online: log on to collegeoftao.com

Shoulder Rotation

Lift your left shoulder and roll it backward, down, forward, and up, making sure to keep your arms relaxed. Repeat three times in each direction. Repeat on your right shoulder. Inhale while circling up and exhale while circling down.

Breathe from the bottom up. Relax, close your eyes for three minutes, and breathe. Like a baby, breathe from low in your abdomen, filling up your lungs from the bottom. Many people breathe primarily from the chest and shoulders, which only worsens feelings of tightness in the upper section of the torso. Breathing from the bottom up will gradually undo this pattern of breathing, and can also help to relieve tension and support a more natural posture. Practice this way of breathing twice daily for two weeks.

Contract and Expand. A quick tension release can be performed by exaggerating the tension before relaxing the muscles. On an inhale, pull your shoulders up high, as close to the ears as possible. Be careful not to overdo it, and stop if you feel any pain. Stretch just enough to feel a moderate pressure. You can emphasize the muscle contraction by squeezing your eyes shut on the same inhale. As you exhale, drop your shoulders, breathe out through an open mouth, and open and relax your eyes. Sense the difference in your neck and shoulders after performing this. You can repeat this several times daily.

Watch online: log on to collegeoftao.com

Elbow Rotation

With your left arm hanging down at your side, place your right hand loosely over the left elbow area. As your left arm moves, it will rub the inside of your right hand. To begin, bend your left arm at the elbow, turning it upwards toward the body while remaining inside your right arm. Continue circling your left forearm away from your body and back down. Repeat three times in both directions. Repeat on right elbow. Inhale while circling up and exhale while circling down.

Watch online: log on to collegeoftao.com

Wrist Rotation

Clasp your hands together with your fingers interlaced. Leading with the thumbs, trace a horizontal figure eight in front of your body with your hands, making sure to maximize the range of motion with your wrists. You can start with a small figure eight and gradually make it larger with each revolution, before reversing the motion to lead with the pinkies, and making the figure eight movements smaller once again. Breathe naturally and deep.

Watch online: log on to collegeoftao.com

Finger Mobilization

This sequence should create a tingling sensation through your hands and fingers. Perform lightly or avoid altogether if this is painful. Repeat tapping several times in each hand position.

- Interlace your fingers, bringing your arms out and in so that the webs of your fingers hit each other. Using a similar motion, tap together the webs between your thumbs and index fingers.
- With your palms up, tap the pinky-side of your hands together. Flip your hands so the palms face down and tap your hands together so the outside of the thumbs and the sides of your index fingers hit each other at the same time.
- Tap the fingertips of your right hand into the palm of the left hand. Repeat this by switching hands.
- Make a loose fist with your right hand and tap it into the palm of your left hand and anywhere else on the hand that needs attention. Repeat by switching hands.
- Give yourself a self massage, using the thumb and first finger of one hand to massage the bones, tendons and muscles of the other hand. Perform on both hands.

Watch online: log on to collegeoftao.com

Hip and Waist Rotation

Start with your feet wide apart (double the width of your shoulders) and legs straight. Place your hands on the sides of your waist. Bend forward at the waist. Keeping your hands in place, turn from the waist and bring your upper body to the left, circling up to standing with a slight back bend, down on the right side, before bending forward again. Repeat three times in both directions. Inhale when circling to the back, exhale when circling to the front.

Hip Rotation

Place the heels together (or farther apart to easily keep balance) with your feet facing forward. Place the palms of your hands over the kidneys on your lower back and rub them several times to warm them up. Keeping your palms over the kidneys and your head positioned over your feet, push your hips forward, then around to the left, behind, to the right, and then forward again. Repeat three times in each direction. Exhale as the hips circle forward, inhale as they circle backward.

Watch online: log on to collegeoftao.com

Back and Core Stretching Exercise

Avoiding a sedentary life is extremely important to keeping your back, and the rest of your body, from experiencing undue pain. Walking, yoga, and Tai Chi are all excellent ways to keep the tissues flexible and the joints nourished and pain-free. If pain has set into your back, try these movements for relief and added strength training:

1.   Stand up straight. Inhale with your chest out and shoulders back. Hold for five seconds. Exhale and repeat.

2.   Lie on your back, with knees bent and your feet flat on the floor. Bring one knee up, then the second, pulling both knees to your chest so the stretch is felt in the buttocks. Bring your forehead to your knees and hold for five seconds. Put your feet down one at a time along with your head. Rest and repeat.

3.   Lie on your back with knees bent and your feet flat on the floor. Inhaling, tighten your buttocks and roll your pelvis upward so your upper back is against the floor. Hold for five seconds. Exhaling, lower your pelvis back down onto the floor. Relax and repeat.

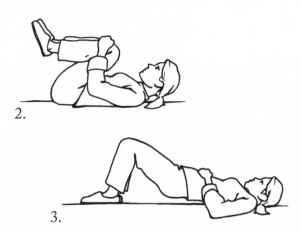

2.

3.

Back Strengthening Exercise

4.   Lie face down with your hands at your sides. Inhaling, lift one leg off the floor. Hold for five seconds while holding your breath. Exhaling, bring your leg down slowly. Rest and repeat on the other side. Alternatively, you can lift your head, shoulders, arms, and legs simultaneously to access more of the muscles in your back.

5.   Move to a kneeling position. Inhaling, arch your back while lowering your head and neck. Hold for five seconds. Exhaling, lower your back while raising your neck and head. Rest and repeat.

Watch online: log on to collegeoftao.com

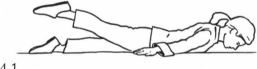

4.1.

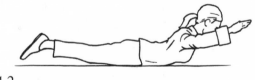

4.2.

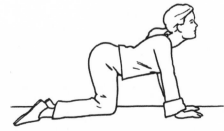

5.

Knee Rotation

With your feet together, bend at the waist to rest your hands on your knees. Gently rub them to warm them up. Keeping your palms centered on the upper ridge of the kneecaps, bend your knees to make a circle, pushing toward your left side, then circling them around in front, to the right side, then straightening back up. Repeat three times in both directions. Next, keeping your knees together, bend them forward and then separate to each side, circling back to center as you straighten your legs. Repeat three times. Reverse the direction of the circles and repeat three more times. Exhale when your knees bend down, inhale when straightening the legs.

Watch online: log on to collegeoftao.com

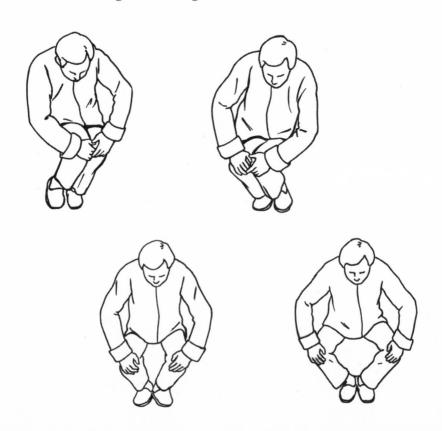

Ankle Rotation

Lift your left foot and rotate it at the ankle three times in both directions. Point and flex the foot, then shake the ankle and the entire leg to loosen the joints. Repeat on your other foot. Your breathing should be deep and natural.

Watch online: log on to <u>collegeoftao.com</u>

Bouncing Your Center

With your feet shoulder width apart, your spine straight and arms hanging loosely by your sides, gently bounce your whole body, focusing on your center of gravity around the pelvis area. The bouncing should start at the balls of your feet and all the joints should be involved in the motion. While most of the movement will come from bending your knees, this motion should elicit a gentle vibration to move the energy to all parts of your body. Sometimes you will bounce vigorously and other times more gently. Follow what your body needs in the moment. This bouncing movement can be performed on its own for a few seconds or up to several minutes at a time when a simple body-wide stimulation, and relaxation, is desired. When completed, take a moment to feel the sensations moving through your body. Vibrating the body in this way has been repeatedly shown to promote bone strength. And when bones are strong, the tissues and joints attached to them are strong as well.

Watch online: log on to collegeoftao.com

Standing Meditation

There are many postures in which to meditate, but standing medita-tion should be the first choice for arthritis sufferers, as in this posi-tion the whole body can be integrated into the practice. The even pressure placed on the joints creates optimal blood flow, allowing for your body's natural pain mediators and cartilage builders to reach the joint without delay.

We recommend that all new students practice two to three minutes every day, gradually working up to five minutes per day, and eventu-ally up to 10 to 15 minutes. Ultimately, this can be performed from a couple minutes to over an hour for those with lots of practice. It's simple and fun. The mind is relaxed, the body is focused, and all of our joints are engaged to maintain this easy posture. We would like to emphasize that this shouldn't be done if pain, extreme fatigue, or dizziness are experienced. Some mild shaking or sweating is normal but will subside with enough practice.

Putting yourself in the position outlined below will take some prac-tice to feel comfortable. At first, this posture will feel different, may-be even uncomfortable. With practice, the spine will be opened al-lowing for fluids and neural messages to flow more freely through the body. Also, maintain a calm and happy mind, focusing more on relaxing and less on the specifics of the movement or meditation be-ing practiced. In time, the details will become second nature to you. Again, start small, just a few minutes and build your time over the weeks. In time the joints will gain strength, the mind will calm, and pain will subside.

Standing Meditation Posture

- Feet are shoulder-width apart, pointing straight forward.
- Knees are slightly bent.
- Your pelvis tilts forward, allowing your tailbone to point straight down, relaxing your lower back by flattening out the curvature.
- Spine is straight.
- Shoulders are relaxed.
- Allow for space under your armpits as you wrap your arms around an imaginary tree trunk in front of you. Turn your palms to face your navel with the fingers pointing toward one another.
- Elbows, wrists, and fingers are relaxed.
- Gently tuck your chin in to allow the vertex of your head to point straight up.
- Place the tip of your tongue on the upper palate just behind your teeth as if saying the letter "N." This connects the two primary channels that run up your spine and down the front of your body.
- Eyes should be slightly open so you are relaxed yet not susceptible to falling asleep.

Meditation Breathing

Your breathing should be slow, smooth, even, and deep. With practice, you can learn to center your breathing set lower in the torso, as if your lungs stretched all the way to your pelvis. Your mind may stay focused on the lower abdomen, feeling warmth and pressure build there with each breath. You can also say the word "calm" to yourself with each exhalation. In this position you may imagine yourself as the light atop a candle. From the great reservoir of Earth energy beneath you, this life force travels unimpeded from the bottom of your feet to the top of your head, emanating from the marrow inside your bones all the way to the surface of your skin; surrounding, filling, and protecting every cell of your body.

You might want to record yourself saying the above steps to start with. This way you can relax and allow the recording to direct you into proper posture, breathing, and intention.

Acupressure Healing

With acupressure you can use a thumb, finger, or blunt object to press and rub a point for local stimulation of the body's healing mechanisms. You can press them on one or both sides of the body. Whichever point is most tender or sore is typically the area to focus on. The few points listed here are for general and specific use.

Where is your pain?

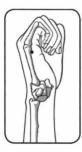

Hands and arms: Winding Gulch (LI-11). Locate this point in the depression at the outer part of the left elbow crease, between the elbow tendon and the bone. The point is best located when the arm is bent at 90 degrees with the palm facing the abdomen. Apply steady pressure with your right thumb until you feel soreness. Hold for 3 minutes. Repeat on the right arm. This helps clear heat and reduce inflammation, as well as detoxify the body.

Feet and legs: Foot Three Mile (ST-36). This acupoint is one of the most important points for tonifying vital energy and blood, as well as promoting general wellness. This point helps regulate digestion and metabolism, calms the mind, and strengthens the body. Find Foot Three Mile four finger-widths below your right knee, on the outside of your kneecap. Apply moderate pressure with your right thumb, and hold for 5 minutes. Repeat on your left leg.

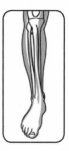

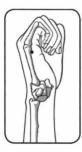

Back/Spine: Back Stream (SI-3). This point is often used to treat pain along the back and the outer parts of the shoulders and arms. This point helps relax and strengthen the tendons, joints, and muscles. With your right hand, make a loose fist. Find this point on the pinkie side of your hand just behind and below the knuckle of your pinkie. Press the point with your left thumb or index finger until you feel soreness. Hold for 3 minutes, and then repeat on your left hand.

Shoulder Pain

It's said that the weight of the world can rest on your shoulders. Stress may find you living with your shoulders raised to your ears, limiting their mobility and predisposing you to pain and tension, especially if there was a previous trauma in that area. Pain in the shoulders that radiates up along the neck is extremely common and can be linked to both emotional tension and excessive use. In urban areas where people tend to drive long distances, or otherwise spend much of their time in cars, the shoulders are prone to hunching even more due to the driving posture - arms outstretched, putting pressure on many of those surrounding structures. The same is true for prolonged computer use and many other activities involving the arms and hands.

Shoulder Acupressure:
Channel Opening (ST-38)

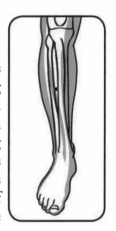

This point relieves pain in the shoulder as well as the lower leg. You can find this point by placing both hands, lining all 10 fingers, below the bottom of your kneecap. Your tenth finger should land in the middle of your shin bone. Channel Opening is located one thumb width outwards from this spot on your shin. To press, place both thumb tips on the point and squeeze your calf with the rest of your hands, pressing for 3 minutes. Repeat on the both sides.

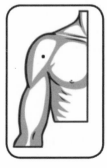

Front of the Shoulder (Jianqian)

This is a tender point on the front of the shoulder. With your right arm relaxed by your side, find this point by starting on the front of the chest at the endpoint of your right armpit crease. From here, the point is less than halfway toward the shoulder bone on the upper and outer part of the shoulder. Find the most tender area and press for 3 minutes with your left thumb. Repeat on the opposite arm.

Neck Pain

At one point or another, almost everyone has woken up with a stiff neck, otherwise known as torticollis. This is often a short-lived strain that goes away on its own within a day or two. But if the strain is severe or if treatment isn't started soon, this relatively simple condition can become a much bigger problem. Imagine having to rotate your whole body to look at something behind you due to a stiff neck. Burning pain, numbness, tingling, and limited range of motion can appear, as well as the whiplash many drivers or athletes may experience. Getting treatment early and often is the key to make sure pain and limited movement are resolved and don't accumulate into full-blown arthritis. Other risk factors for the neck area include colds and flus along with the characteristic neck stiffness (often accompanied by whole body aches, pains, and stiffness). Windy climates can also predispose some to chronic neck pain and immobility.

Neck Acupressure

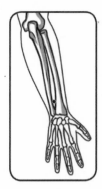

Outer Gate (SJ-5)

This point is used for pain in the wrist, but also pain in the shoulders, neck, and outer arms and elbows. This point can be found two thumb-widths above your wrist on the outside of your right arm, in between the two tendons. Apply pressure with your left thumb until you find a sore spot. Hold for 3 minutes and then repeat on your left arm.

Wind Pond (GB-20)

Often prescribed for headaches and neck pain, this point will also help harmonize your immune system. This point is found in the natural indentation at the base of your skull on both sides of your neck. With your thumbs, press and lift up toward the base of your skull and lean your head back. Use the weight of your head against your thumbs for a steady pressure. Hold for about 5 minutes. Breathe deeply and slowly during the acupressure.

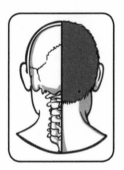

Back Pain

Most people will experience some sort of back pain during their life. But if you suffer from chronic back or spinal pain, you should have a thorough checkup to discover the origin of your pain. The most common causes of back pain include excessive physical work, excessive sexual activity, pregnancy and childbirth, incorrect or inadequate exercise, exposure to cold and damp conditions, and not enough rest. If any of these scenarios go unchecked, osteoarthritis of the spine may appear at any of joints that connect the vertebrae. Many types of back pain respond well to acupuncture and herbal treatments. Arthritis of the spine, however, may not be the only source of chronic back pain. Other things like slipped disks or even infection can cause back pain, too. On the other hand, severe degenerative arthritis can also develop with little to no pain, so make sure your case is completely reviewed to best manage your expectations. If there are no signs of heat (red, swollen areas or a burning feeling) then a heating pad, warm bath, or heat lamp can relax the tissues while stimulating blood circulation and energy to relieve the pain.

Back Acupressure

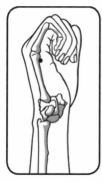

Back Stream (SI-3)

This point is often used to treat pain along the back and the outer parts of the shoulders and arms. This point helps relax and strengthen the tendons, joints, and muscles. With your right hand, make a loose fist. Find this point on the pinkie side of your hand just behind and below the knuckle of your pinkie. Press the point with your left thumb or index finger until you feel soreness. Hold for 3 minutes, and then repeat on your left hand.

Hundred Meeting (DU-20)

This point is on top of your head, midway between your ears. Apply steady pressure with your index finger until you feel a sore spot, and hold for 3 minutes.

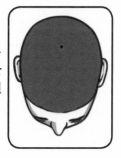

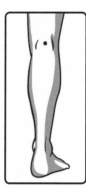

Balance The Core (UB-40)

This point is good for strengthening the kidneys and alleviating back and knee pain. Find this point in the middle of the crease behind your right knee. Use your right middle finger to apply pressure until you feel a slight soreness. Then hold for 3 minutes, and repeat on your left leg.

Elbow Pain

These joints can present with adjacent tendonitis associated with playing tennis, playing golf, repetitive lifting, or excessive work. The joint itself can become arthritic if over-taxed with these or similar activities. Acupressure on Winding Gulch (LI11) is arguably the most important local point for elbow pain.

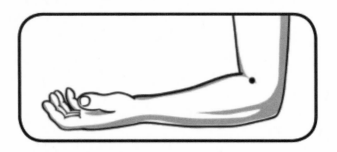

Elbow Acupressure:

Winding Gulch (LI-11)

Locate this point in the depression at the outer part of the left elbow crease, between the elbow tendon and the bone. The point is best located when the arm is bent at 90 degrees with the palm facing the abdomen. Apply steady pressure with your right thumb until you feel soreness. Hold for 3 minutes. Repeat on the right arm. This helps clear heat and reduce inflammation, as well as detoxify the body.

Hand and Finger Pain

Almost everything we do requires the use of our fingers. The many joints that link our fingers together can suffer from both osteoarthritis, which results from overuse, and rheumatoid arthritis, which results from a faulty autoimmune response.

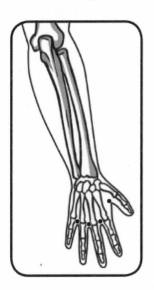

Finger Acupressure:
Eight Pathogens (Ba Xie)

These points clear inflammation and swelling in the hand and are also used for headaches. These eight points are found when fists are made, finding them halfway between the back of the hand and the ends of the creases between the fingers. Press the points on the left hand with the thumb or first finger of the right hand. Hold each for 3 minutes. Repeat on the right hand.

Wrist Pain

Excess use or over flexing/extending can predispose your wrists to pain. Carpal tunnel syndrome may easily be confused with arthritis, but if left untreated the compromised movement due to pain can make any existing arthritis that much more difficult to treat. Carpal tunnel syndrome is the inflammation of a band of tissue that holds in all the nerves and blood vessels that pass through the wrist. Directly underneath the skin is a wide bracelet-sized band that, if inflamed, can make wrist movement very painful.

Wrist Acupressure

Outer Gate (SJ-5)

This point is used for pain in the wrist, but also pain in the shoulders and outer arms and elbows. This point can be found two thumb-widths above your wrist on the outside of your right arm, in between the two tendons. Apply pressure with your left thumb until you find a sore spot. Hold for 3 minutes and then repeat on your left arm.

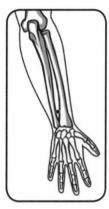

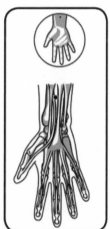

Inner Gate (P-6)

This acupoint is often used to harmonize the stomach and relieve nausea and vomiting as well as alleviate pain on the inside of the wrist and arm. Find Inner Gate three finger-widths above your wrist crease, between the two tendons on the inside of your right forearm. Apply moderate pressure with your left thumb. Hold for 5 minutes, and then repeat on your other arm.

Carpal Tunnel Test. You can test your level of inflammation by using the prayer or reversed-prayer hand positions. To test the inner wrist, place your forearms parallel to the ground in front of your chest with your palms pressed together and fingers pointing upward. Healthy tissue should sustain this posture pain-free for at least 30 seconds. To test the outer wrist, which is more often the site of pain, simply place the back of the hands together in this same arm position with the fingers pointing downward. Test for the same amount of time.

Hip Pain

Hip health is crucial to maintaining a long, healthy life. This is the site of the largest joint in the body, which connects the femur, the largest bone in the body, to the pelvis. Pain located here can limit our ability to walk; and if osteoporosis is an issue, arthritic pain can make it difficult to put a stop to bone loss. A lack of proper exercise is one of the main factors contributing to bone loss, and with added arthritic pain people may become even less motivated to exercise, which only makes the joint pain and bone loss that much worse. At later ages, a break in the hip due to bone loss requires significant bed rest and usually accounts for a reduction in lifespan. This downward spiral should be avoided if possible. Of the more than 200,000 total hip replacement surgeries performed in the U.S. every year, most of them are in people over 60 years old. If issues in the hip are chronic, a combination of treatments is usually called for, as one modality is usually not enough to effect relief.

Hip Acupressure:

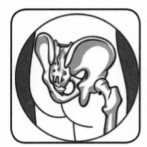

Jumping Circle (GB-30)

This point benefits both the hips and legs, and is useful for relieving pain. This point is also good for relaxing and strengthening the tendons. This acupoint is located on the center of your buttocks about midway between the tip of your tailbone and left hipbone. Apply heavy pressure with your thumb or by leaning against a tennis ball until you feel soreness. Hold for 30 seconds and release. Repeat several times, alternating from the left hip to the right.

Extending Vessel (UB-62)

This point is useful for outer ankle pain but is often used for headache and pain in the back of the neck, spine, and hips as well. Find this point on your right ankle, moving downward from the outer ankle bone until you find the soft tissue, about 2 thumb widths below. Press with your right thumb for 3 minutes and repeat on the other side.

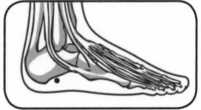

Foot and Toe Pain

Most often, the issue here is gout. While typically felt in the big joint on the big toe, gout can strike many other joints of the foot or body. The red, hot, swollen, painful joint is due to a buildup of uric acid crystals that grind away at the joints and surrounding tissues. When dealing with goat, it's best to avoid sugar, alcohol, meat, and seafood. Use an icepack for twenty minutes several times a day to treat the pain and inflammation. Once gone, weight management, nutrition, and regular exercise are important tools to keep symptoms from returning. Similar symptoms can also arise from consuming foods rich in oxalic acid. In this case, it's not true gout. Foods to avoid include spinach, chard, and chives. Commonly, osteoarthritis and rheumatoid arthritis can strike the toes as well.

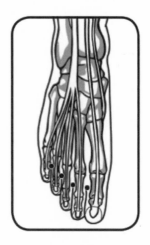

Toe Acupressure:
Eight Winds (Bafeng)
These 8 points clear inflammation and swelling of the toes and are also useful for headache and irregular periods. Find each of these points between the toes, at half a thumb-width upward from the ends of each toe crease. Press with the thumb or first finger on each point for 3 minutes.

Ankle Pain

Overuse is a big issue when it comes to your ankle joints, and they are a frequent site of sprains. This is the first major joint that our body weight rests on, and the health of this joint can ripple its beneficial effects to the rest of the body. There is a Chinese saying that states, "People get sick from the ankles up." In other words, once the ankles' mobility and health is in question, it becomes more difficult to properly move and care for the rest of your body.

Ankle Acupressure:

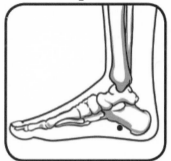

<u>Shining Sea (K-6)</u>
Shining Sea is useful for inner ankle pain but also helps with insomnia, frequent urination, and throat disorders like pain, swelling, or dryness. Find this point on the left ankle by sliding the left thumb downward from the inner ankle bone until you feel the soft tissue beneath the ankle, approximately 2 thumb widths below. Press for 3 minutes and repeat on the right foot with the right thumb.

<u>Extending Vessel (UB-62)</u>
This point is useful for outer ankle pain but is often used for headache and pain in the back of the neck, spine, and hips as well. Find this point on your right ankle, moving downward from the outer ankle bone until you find the soft tissue, about 2 thumb widths below. Press with your right thumb for 3 minutes and repeat on the other side.

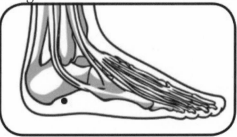

Knee Pain

Knees are a very exposed and easily injured part of the body, and frequently suffer from overuse. Old knee injuries often return as joint pain later in life. Sudden pain or swelling that appears on only one knee is more of a local issue and can be treated quickly with acupuncture and herbal medicine. But if both knees are affected by a pain that slowly increases over time, this can point to a more systemic weakness, one that calls for an evaluation of the whole body. Partial or total knee replacement surgery can often be called for, either when the patient suffers from severe arthritic degeneration, or when all other therapies have been exhausted. About 270,000 of these surgeries are performed annually in the U.S. Undergoing this surgery comes with its own complications as well as a long recovery time, so in addition to working with your acupuncturist for pre- and post-operative care, always get a thorough evaluation from at least two orthopedists if surgery is recommended.

Knee Acupressure

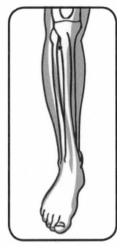

<u>Foot Three Mile (ST-36)</u>
This acupoint is one of the most important points for tonifying vital energy and blood, as well as promoting general wellness. This point helps regulate digestion and metabolism, calms the mind, and strengthens the body. Find Foot Three Mile four finger-widths below your right knee, on the outside of your kneecap. Apply moderate pressure with your right thumb, and hold for 5 minutes. Repeat on your left leg.

<u>Yin Mound Spring (SP-9)</u>
Yin Mound Spring is often used for swelling and pain in the knee but also helps digestive disorders including diarrhea and abdominal pain. Find this point by running your right thumb on the inside of your right shin bone, gliding upward in a straight line along the soft tissue until your motion is stopped by the bottom of your knee. Press here for 3 minutes and repeat on the left side.

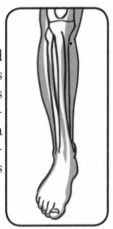

Chapter Five:
Your Mind, Stress
and Inflammation

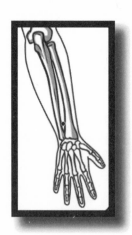

Am I Making Myself Worse?

Have you ever found that after a prolonged stressful or emotional event you find yourself with more pain in your body? I think most people would agree that the connection between emotional and physical pain is a nearly universal experience. Studies also confirm the link between the mind and the body, especially in fields like psychoneuroimmunology where the effects of negative thoughts, mental disorders, and stress on the immune systems are well documented. Your personality can also play into the development of arthritis. There are three characteristics that seem to make patients more prone to arthritis: negative self-criticism, resistance to change, and rigidity in lifestyle. Your ability to accept your current reality, share your feelings, and be open to change will take you a long way on your journey to recovery. There are numerous techniques that you can learn and practice that will help your emotional stability and also promote a beneficial outcome for your illness. They include meditation, affirmation, and building a supportive community of family and friends. By recognizing the potential mental and emotional factors that may contribute to your illness and by utilizing helpful techniques, you will be able to assist in your own healing process and have more joy and fulfillment in your life.

Your Mind Triggers Physical Inflammation

Emotions are a normal part of life. But when one or more emotions become a constant strain on the mind, physical symptoms can develop. Whether it is anger, sadness, excitement, worry, or fear, our emotions serve a purpose. They keep our internal energies moving. But when an emotion becomes suppressed or over-expressed, problems can result. In Chinese medicine, emotional suppression such as repressed anger or over-expression like excess worry is seen as energetic stagnation. When energy stagnates, it can create swelling, heat or cold, and pain. This can also limit circulation of vital nutrients and expulsion of toxins and waste products. This, in turn, can cause inflammation, which if prolonged, leads to degeneration and breakdown of tissue.

The human body responds to physical and emotional threats in similar ways, by triggering the release of immune proteins that hasten wound repair and reduce infection. These proteins are called inflammatory cytokines and are useful in healing from acute injury. However, frequent activation of the immune system over time due to stress triggers and the brain's perception of danger will increase the risk of all kinds of inflammatory diseases like rheumatoid arthritis, asthma, and heart disease. Since your body can't differentiate between a real or perceived threat, what your mind perceives as dangerous will translate into physical response. It is therefore imperative to be mindful of your feelings and examine how you respond to stressful situations in order to prevent making yourself sick.

Soothe Your Nerves with Sound Healing

In Chinese medicine, the nervous system correlates to the liver system, so nervousness, depression and anxiety can be balanced by working through the liver. A traditional technique to soothe the nerves is the practice of healing sounds. Simply saying "Shh" as you exhale engages the energies in the liver and the nervous system, as well as in the network of tendons and ligaments. Slowly inhale through the nose, then exhale while saying the "Shh" sound as if you were calmly telling someone to be quiet. Imagine any pain or emotional tension flowing out of your body and into the ground. Practice the healing sound a minimum of 12 times. You can do this as often as you like. I recommend doing it once a day for no less than two weeks. If you toss and turn at night or have an overactive mind that keeps you from sleeping soundly, you can also do this exercise right before bed. You may be surprised by the calming effects of the healing sounds and how they help you to increase your energy and lessen your pain.

Share What Ails Thee

One basic, universal truth is this: you are not alone. Many people share the same experiences as you, such as disease, relationship challenges, financial woes, or emotional hardships. When challenged with pain or immobility some people choose to close themselves off emotionally, or even physically, from those around them. But by doing so, you only serve to keep your potential help away from you. Try to practice reaching out and asking for help by sharing your experiences, both good and bad, with your friends and loved ones. Not only will it help to ease your mind, but you may find that your body responds as well. One study found much improvement in people with rheumatoid arthritis who were in supportive relationships. Join a local arthritis support group or simply get out and engage more with the caring people in your community. The internet is full of places to look for more ideas on activities and groups to join. Share and lighten the load and you'll be better for it.

Cultivate Positive Beliefs Within Yourself

Words like "faith" and "belief" hold strong meanings for many people. Your faith in the success of each step along the way in the process of healing will surely make an impact on your recovery. Some medical professionals will say that belief has no bearing on the outcome of a medical procedure, but it has been documented that faith can activate physical healing. Putting ideas of faith aside for a moment, consider what a medical procedure would be like if you were certain it was going to help you. If you knew without a doubt that the acupuncture, massage, or nutritional program was going to fix the problem well before even beginning your treatment, what would that feel like? Take one minute right now to close your eyes and feel with your mind how that process could be for you. Picture yourself walking into the softly lit treatment center, confidently shaking the hand of the practitioner that's going to change your life, looking in his or her eyes and saying, "I trust you" and "Thank you." Feel that part of your body being cared for by a team of people, compassionately removing your blockages of pain and frustration. Finally, see yourself walking out of the treatment center and into your home, feeling healed, satisfied, and better than before. This is positive thinking in action. It will lift your mood and your outlook. It will help. It is rather difficult to stay depressed when you're wearing a perfect smile, and positive thinking is like smiling with your mind.

You Are Not Your Car

I have a patient who says, "Every time I get out of my car my back hurts." I asked, "What kind of car do you drive?" I learned she drove a small, two-seater sports car. I inquired, "Did you consider getting a different car?" She replied, "Well, that wouldn't be me." My patient was so attached to her image that she didn't recognize that she was unnecessarily torturing herself by contorting her spine while getting into and out of a car that didn't suit her body. She was no longer just driving, she was rolling her ego around in a little cage on wheels. High heels are another instance of the physical price of fashion. The feet are bound, the toes smashed together and the heels elevated. High heels were designed with ballerinas in mind, with tall, slender, sensual legs in mind. But this singular invention, worn by many women, is responsible for countless cases of pain and deformity of the lower extremities. Arthritis can be seen as a limitation placed on how you move and express yourself. Pain sufferers want to free themselves from such restriction. Part of this freedom comes from the ability to transcend the ego and let go of who you think you are. What you wear and what you drive may contribute to a false sense of self. Look at yourself and your life. See what you're doing in each moment. Discover if you are, in fact, creating your own pain and decide if that pain is worth the choices you make.

Do You Have the Personality for Arthritis?

It is well established that Type A personalities (those that are impatient, competitive, and hard charging) are more likely to suffer from heart disease, high blood pressure, and strokes. On the other hand, people with Type B personalities are analytical, deliberate, and methodical. According to a large study, Type B personalities are almost 75% less likely to develop job-related injuries and diseases than Type A people. Arthritis sufferers tend to exhibit excessive self-criticism, resistance to change, and rigidity in lifestyle. Many people are resigned to the personality that they are "born with," and argue that they cannot change their predisposition, as if their personality were a matter of genetics. It is almost like saying that personality is predestined, and therefore we should just live with the consequences that it brings. In reality, this could not be further from the truth. You can change your personality if you want to, as soon as you choose to stop being a victim of your own habits. Choose to discover which aspect of your personality isn't serving you and make a decision to change it today. Start by writing down which trait you want to change. Be aware of it each time before you express it and give yourself two minutes of "time-out" before you respond. For example, if you are prone to reacting with anger and want to change that response, become aware of circumstances that tend to trigger your angry reactions and give yourself two minutes before dealing with the situation. Most likely, your negative emotional impulse will have dissipated by then.

Let Go of Rigidity

A rigid lifestyle or a rigid mind can literally create a rigid body. The stiffness in our muscles, tendons, and joints can be a product of our constricted lifestyle or our inflexible attachment to certain ideas. These ideas can include the way we see ourselves, the way we spend our free time, or the way we interact with other people. Many of these habits aren't conscious to us. However, once you consciously acknowledge that you are experiencing pain, or a disease, or something "wrong" with you, you have the chance to search for the factors that have contributed to this undesirable state. The simple task of looking inward for a solution is a good start, and the best way to produce lasting relief. Look at your relationships. Are your expectations of yourself or other people unrealistic? Look at your schedule. Have you left any time to have fun or take care of yourself or your family? Look at your whole body. Has a recent health concern concealed another, older issue you've been ignoring? Do you hold tension in your neck, shoulders, back, hips, or stomach? Look at your mind. Do you find yourself thinking so much that it's hard to focus, to sleep, or to relax? When you find something you feel interferes with your health, start experimenting with new ways to replace it. If you've been trying something for a while without success, it might be time for something else. Try to add a little spontaneity to your usual routines to break up your habits and let go of rigidity.

Flexible Mind, Flexible Body

Bamboo is prized in Asia, not only for the use of its sprouts as food, its inner stem as medicine, and its stalk as construction material, but also for its cultural significance as a symbol of flexibility. The supple plant is able to survive even the most devastating storms. Our lives, too, are filled with unexpected happenings, and those of us who are successful at adapting to change are healthier and more fulfilled. Studies from China have shown that patients who possess flexibility as a personality trait often recover from illnesses 50 percent faster than those who cling stubbornly to their tired habits. Try not to become overly attached to a specific outcome. Stay on the course you have charted for your life, but understand that when barriers present themselves, sometimes you need to take a detour in order to get back on track. Practice stretching, yoga, or Tai Chi. Being physically flexible can encourage the same trait in your personality.

Meditate, Don't Medicate

For thousands of years, meditation has been practiced in the East as a tool for inner peace and spirituality. There are as many meditation techniques as there are traditions. In most techniques, the discipline involves the practice of breathing and visualization methods. The effects of regular meditation have been well documented. Some benefits include lowered blood pressure, a decreased risk of heart disease, decreased chronic pain, and increased mental clarity. Often, it only requires fifteen minutes of practice daily to enjoy the health benefits of meditation.

Try this simple meditation to release tension. While sitting or lying down, focus on letting go of the tension in every part of your body, moving from the head down to the toes. Take one breath for the head, and one for the neck. Next, one breath each for the back, shoulders, arms, elbows, hands, chest, back, stomach, hips, thighs, knees, calves, ankles, feet, and toes. Each time you exhale, feel the stress and stiffness melt away as you say to yourself, "calm." After you've released the tension in your whole body, focus on the bottom of your feet for 3 minutes. You can repeat this as many times as you like until you feel completely relaxed. For a detailed and guided meditation experience, please try the *Meditation for Stress Release* CD. Start meditating today and feel your tension begin to melt away. See the Resources section for more information.

Stress Can Be an "Inside Job"

Stress is usually caused by an external stimulus, but our responses play a big role in how it will affect us. Consider the study of two groups of mice in which one group was exposed to a live cat outside their cages, and the other was exposed to an identical toy cat. The group of mice exposed to the live cat developed more diseases and lived only a third as long as the toy cat group. The mice in the toy cat group were apparently able to figure out that there was no real danger from the toy cat and eventually simply ignored it. By re-framing our perspective on stressful situations, we can often see that the danger is largely an illusion. When we moderate our reactions to potential stressors, we too can neutralize negative situations.

Invocation for Health and Longevity

The power of our intentions can create a physical response, as proven by biofeedback and mind-body research. It can also elicit energetic responses from the divine universe. Traditionally, an invocation is a verse recited aloud or silently with mental and spiritual intent focused on a beneficial outcome. From the Taoist longevity tradition, I will share with you this Invocation for Health and Longevity:

I am strong; the sky is clear. I am strong; the earth is solid. I am strong; humans are at peace with one another. My life is supported by the harmonious spheres of body, mind, and spirit within my being. All of my spiritual elements return to me. All of my spiritual guardians accompany me. The yin and yang of my being are well integrated. My life is firmly rooted. As I follow the path of revitalization, my mind and emotions become wholesome and active. The goddess of my heart nourishes my life abundantly. Internal energy balances my spiritual growth and all obstacles dissolve before me. My natural healing power contributes to a long and happy life, so that my virtuous fulfillment in the world can be accomplished. By following the subtle law and integral way of life, I draw ever closer to the divine source of health and longevity.

See the Resources section for more information.

Accepting Your Condition

You're likely reading this book to educate yourself and look for ways to improve your health. Reversing pain and improving your well-being are honorable goals. However, there is another aspect to healing that should not be overlooked: acceptance of your current state. This doesn't mean you should give up or ignore your disease. Rather, it means that healing tends to happen more completely when the body and mind are at peace. Being at ease with your condition will only help. It can be exasperating to be constantly looking for the magic bullet, for treatments that will permanently cure your disease once and for all, returning you to the life you knew before all this started. While this is certainly possible with acute diseases, it is less so with chronic, degenerative conditions like arthritis. Conditions that take time to develop will also take time to repair. Healing isn't always a linear experience. In order to change anything you must accept where you are in your reality right now, no matter how bleak it may appear. Make the best of the current situation, because it's not going to be the same forever. Nothing ever is. You may be surprised to find, once you open up to the positive qualities of your condition, that there is something to be learned from it. There are always opportunities for growth when confronted with challenge or discomfort.

Try saying this aloud: *"I accept my condition. Right now, I feel pain. That is all it is – a feeling. All of my experiences, including my disease, are part of me right now and I accept them all. I know it will not be like this forever. My life is full of so much more than this one feeling. I am open to what the rest of my life will bring."*

For more guidance, consider working with a wellness coach or therapist.

Cooling Inflammation with Detox Meditation

This practice is good for any kind of pain, but it works especially well for joint pain with visible redness or feelings of burning or warmth. Start by closing your eyes while sitting or lying down. Breathe through your nose, slow and deep from the belly. Guide your mental intention as a beam of light, focusing on the area of pain or blockage. See this area turn into a dense, cold block of ice. See and feel the energetic state of this tissue. Using your beam of light, on an exhale, see this ice block melt into cold water surrounding and penetrating this area. On another exhale, see this water melt into a fine, cold mist. When this blocked, painful area has completely dissolved into cold air, exhale this toxic mist out of your body, feeling this energetic waste leave you and falling deep into the center of the earth. Repeat this cycle as many times as needed, using your beam of light to transform this problem area from ice, to water, to mist, over and over again. Continue until all pain, blockages, and toxins are released from the body, leaving you in a state of peace and balance. To end, place your hands over one another below your navel. As you breathe, focus your intention on your lower abdomen as your breath fills your center with restorative energy. Try practicing this daily for at least 15 minutes for a minimum of two weeks to see results.

CHAPTER FIVE | 191

A Skeptic Becomes a Convert with Meditation

A patient of ours, who sits for long hours every day at his job and is frequently under severe stress, came in for a series of treatments. Over time his prolonged sitting at work created a very uncomfortable feeling of heat and pain in the muscles around his ischium (otherwise known as the hip bones). He had never tried meditation before, and when we began, he was very skeptical that meditating would do him any physical good. But after just a few short minutes of focusing on a relaxed intention to melt his discomfort away, he was pleasantly surprised to note a complete absence of the heat and pain that had been surrounding his joints. He quickly became a convert and was motivated to continue this simple meditation practice regularly, which was instrumental in a substantial improvement of his arthritic condition.

Positive Emotions Increase Healing

Survivors of personal tragedies, natural disasters, and concentration camps have attributed their survival to hope, optimism, and perseverance. Many studies have been conducted on positive emotions and their impact on health, wellbeing, and healing. These emotions include optimism, hope, serenity, joy and laughter. When subjects were provoked to experience optimism and hope, their levels of cortisol decreased and their endorphins increased. Cortisol is a stress hormone that is often implicated in inflammation, whereas endorphins are associated with pain relief and a calm state of mind. Moreover, when rheumatoid arthritis subjects were asked to experience 30 minutes of laughter daily, there were markedly lower pro-inflammatory cytokines and an increase in anti-inflammatory cytokines. In other words, RA patients experienced an improvement in their condition when laughter was incorporated into their daily life, which is proof that happier people are healthier and better able to heal.

Chapter Six:
Integrative Healing

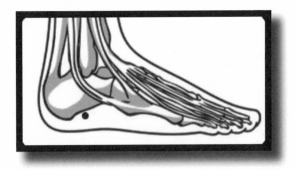

We are entering a new era of health care where the patient and the practitioner work together as a team, sharing the responsibility for their wellness and recovery. There will always be the promise of a quick fix, but people are gradually recognizing that simply taking a pill to make all their problems go away isn't very realistic, nor is it always effective. In the West we make our doctors responsible for healing us. In the East the patient is responsible for their own health and they look to their doctors to guide them on the road to recovery. When patients take responsibility for their own well-being and allow their doctors to provide not just treatment but also guidance on how to participate in their healing process, the outcome is often far superior.

Who is Responsible For My Health?

In the U.S. doctors are responsible for patient records, but in China the patient is responsible for their own paperwork and medical records. Not only does this ensure everyone on their medical team has access to the same information, but it puts patients in a crucially central role in caring for themselves. In the West we often say, "I get sick," as if it came from somewhere else. The equivalent phrase is Chinese is, "I produce disease." As you can see, there are cultures that closely link a disorder to one's ability to manage their own lifestyle and wellness. We are not suggesting you avoid professional help when you get sick, but ignoring your own intuitive ability to know your body on a deeper level may not only slow the healing process but may even be the cause of many common illnesses.

This book introduces a whole new medical system from China, where more than a billion citizens benefit from Chinese medicine every day. This system is rooted in a different paradigm than Western medicine. It emphasizes responsibility on the patient's part, while the doctors' role is discovering and treating the root of the illness with modalities like acupuncture, body work, physical therapy, nutritional and herbal remedies, and counseling to first support the body's natural healing abilities before intervening with modalities like drugs, injections, and surgeries. The goal is to move from the least invasive to the most invasive, encouraging collaboration between East and West treatments for the ultimate benefit of the patient. Engaging patients in proactive and preventive measures by helping them to make lifestyle, dietary, and emotional/spiritual changes puts the control back with the person who matters the most—you! Ask your healthcare provider for information on how to be proactive in your care. In the meantime, consult the resources detailed in this book to address the common complaints of patients managing and living with arthritis.

Root and Branch of Illness

There is a concept in Chinese Medicine called *Root and Branch*. A tree is made up of many parts, growing from the root and spreading its body all the way to the farthest-reaching branches. Pain is often said to be a symptomatic branch. When this problematic branch has been cut off with a painkiller, it's only the branch that's momentarily gone. The rest of the tree, or health problem, still resides under the surface, growing more problem branches all the time. Once symptomatic relief is achieved it's time to go after the root, tackling the whole problematic tree. Whether the solution is treatment by itself, or making changes to the way we live and perceive our lives, some amount of change is needed to address the underlying cause, or root, that manifested the pain in the first place. Addressing these underlying root causes may mean receiving treatment for seemingly unrelated problems. For example, someone suffering from intestinal inflammation may also have arthritic pain. In order to heal the arthritis pain, which is the branch, the root problem in the digestive tract must be extinguished. Remember, your body is a living network and most things happening inside your body are connected in some way.

Wellness Care is More Than Prevention

Once pain and other symptoms are relieved (those pesky branches) and the underlying causes are under control (the problematic roots), wellness care can begin. This includes the ability to remain mindful of what the original problem was and the commitment to continue treating the issue on a consistent, though less-regular basis than when treating the acute pain. This type of preventative care has served a primary role in Traditional Chinese Medicine for thousands of years. A classic Chinese proverb illustrates the point well, "If one waits until they are thirsty before digging a well or until war is upon them before forging weapons, is this not too late?"

Chinese medicine believes in taking care of problems while they are small, so everyday allergies, muscle strains, colds and flus, diarrhea, and headaches are taken seriously by practitioners of acupuncture and Chinese medicine. Even in the absence of symptoms a practitioner can detect subtle changes in your body and mind before a problem arises and advise you with solutions to prevent its onset. Going beyond prevention, a good practitioner will also formulate a plan to help you achieve your full health and longevity potential.

Taking Charge of Your Healing Choices

Whether you see an acupuncturist, a conventional medical doctor, a physical therapist, or a combination of the three, it is important to build a team of professionals to support you in determining the best solution for your condition. After you've been educated on your disorder and your treatment options, you're left to decide how to proceed. Maybe you will find that acupuncture is what offers you the relief and rehabilitation you're looking for, or you may discover that herbal therapy and surgery are what makes sense for your situation. No amount of searching the internet or reviewing statistics will take the place of working directly with medical professionals to create a path to health in which you can place your trust. But part of your journey will always include having you in the driver's seat, because you are ultimately responsible for your health and wellbeing. This means educating yourself, asking the right questions, and holding yourself accountable for your own decisions.

Healing Requires Patience

Speed isn't everything. There's a classic story that demonstrates the difference between Western medicine and Chinese medicine, saying that when attempting to fix a "sick" table, the former is a saw and the latter is a file. The table's "disease" was that it had lost its original circular shape and acquired corners, becoming square in shape. The table sought help from the MD, who quickly took out the saw and hacked off the corners, but in the process nicked one of the legs. The corners were gone, but the circular shape the table once knew wasn't exactly right. Its corners were now something between the two previous shapes, and it looked somewhat ragged. Its leg had also been damaged and would never look or feel the same.

A different table, suffering the same affliction, visited a doctor of Chinese medicine instead. The doctor closely inspected the corners, the tabletop, the legs, and its attachments, in order to familiarize himself with the construction and quality of the whole table before beginning any treatment. After making his assessment, the doctor pulled out a file and began to meticulously whittle down the corners. The table had to return to the Chinese doctor several times because the treatment was comparatively slower. But in the end, the table's shape was restored without incurring any side effects.

This story points out that while quick relief is important, doing it right the first time, regardless of speed, could prove more crucial to your pain relief in the long run. Incremental, progressive change that heals deeper and broader could be the turtle that wins the race when compared to the swift rabbit.

Holistic Paradigm of Acupuncture

Picture the earth in your mind. We know that all our oceans are connected, which means that if one ocean is dirty then all oceans will be affected. The seafood we eat contains varying levels of heavy metals and toxins due to the pollution building up on our planet, especially in the groundwater. The human body's internal ecosystem isn't much different from the makeup of the Earth. Like the earth, we're made of about 70% water. When circulation is poor in one part of the body, the whole body is affected. A doctor of acupuncture and Chinese medicine will always inspect and look at a disease's effect on the entire body rather than just the parts that hurt. Arthritis, like many other conditions, frequently exists alongside other active diseases. More than half of the 23.6 million Americans diagnosed with diabetes also suffer from arthritis, and the majority of those with heart disease have joint pain as well. Taking care of the arthritis by itself usually isn't enough for patients like these. Chinese medicine has long recognized that the body is a connected whole and that an imbalance in one system will surely affect other systems. That's why acupuncture uses acupoints on adjoining meridians that are connected to one another. In other words, we seek to treat diabetes, heart disease, and arthritis all at the same time, as they are all related conditions with the same underlying cause.

A Medicine Customized Just for You

Traditional Chinese Medicine is a system of healing based on an ancient naturalistic philosophy with more than 5,000 years of practice and refinement. Chinese medicine employs the body's own healing mechanisms and is effective for many physical and emotional conditions. Prevention and longevity are the founding principles of Chinese medicine. It is useful for relieving pain, preventing illness, and supporting a healthy lifestyle. The body and mind are treated as an integrated whole, and the focus is on treating the person rather than the disease. Humans are complex creatures made of cells, thoughts, emotions, fluids, and processes that require constant care and attention to stay healthy. Acupuncture, bodywork therapies, nutrition, and herbal medicines are all customized by a practitioner to meet the unique needs of each patient. There isn't a one-size-fits-all treatment for everyone. However, many people suffering from chronic arthritis fail to get customized treatments unique to them. But if you have been unsuccessful in finding relief with what you've tried so far, Chinese medicine may have just the solution you've been searching for.

Acupuncture Removes Blockages to Self-Healing

In ancient China, people observed the phenomenon of a universal life energy they called Qi (pronounced "chi") that circulated throughout every living being along pathways in the body. Health was maintained if this energy flowed freely, but when the pathways were blocked and the Qi no longer flowed smoothly, it resulted in pain and disease. Imagine body fluids stagnating like a swamp or the nervous system short-circuiting; these are symptoms of Qi blockages and causes of disease. Acupuncture was invented more than five millennia ago to address these very blockages and guide your body back to doing what it does best. The art of acupuncture is in the placement of fine needles along defined pathways, stimulating a focused response from the nervous, cardiovascular, musculoskeletal, hormonal, and immune systems, restoring Qi movement and bringing balance and harmony back to the body. Arthritic pain and inflammation respond well to acupuncture and many studies have confirmed its efficacy. You can expect an average case of arthritic pain to improve after only a few treatments. But if the arthritic condition is more severe or long-lasting, it may take a longer course of treatments, more than 10 or 12, before progress can be noticed.

204 | Arthritis: Secrets of Natural Healing

The Miraculous Needle

Acupuncture has been used to effectively treat everything from the symptoms of the common cold to side effects from chemotherapy. But how, exactly, does it work? Conventional understanding is focused primarily on the nervous, circulatory, and hormonal systems. When an acupuncturist inserts very fine needles under the skin, mast cells throughout the skin release chemicals which instantly produce leukotrienes. Leukotrienes are molecules that dilate the small blood vessels in the local area, allowing white blood cells to exit the vessels and reduce the local inflammation, relieving pain. Mast cells also produce prostaglandins, hormone-like substances that communicate with the adjacent nerves. This added rush of prostaglandins informs the brain that it hasn't been doing enough to subdue the pain and, thanks to the acupuncture needle's effect, the brain releases endorphins from the mid-brain as well as from the blood vessels close to the site of pain. Endorphins are the body's most powerful pain-relieving substances, and they are able to block pain receptors along the spine and at the site of pain. Endorphins are also the source of the relaxed state one feels after a session of acupuncture.

Acupuncture needles are often inserted at the site of pain, but they may also be introduced at acupoints far from the affected part of your body. Patients rightly question, "Why are you putting needles in my right elbow if my left knee hurts?" This is another example of how the body is a living network; stimulate one area and the rest of the organism responds. An acupuncture needle is nothing more than a sliver of stainless steel. Truly, it is the truly miraculous human body, with its inherent will to live and cure itself, which deserves all the credit in healing. The needle, in response to stimuli ranging from food, people, activity, emotion, and environment that the body is exposed to, sends a signal to the brain and the rest of the body to activate healing. Acupuncture and Chinese medicine are the clinical applications of this powerful natural response inherent within you.

Herbal Therapy Supports Healthy Functions

Chinese herbs have several unique properties and functions, most of which work to nourish your body. They provide a function similar to vegetables, in that they support the healthy functional of your body's organ systems, but the benefits derived from herbs are much more intense. Herbal therapy works in tandem with acupuncture and provides nutritional support, restores balance, and promotes lasting relief. Once the type of arthritis has been determined, your doctor will create a personalized formula for you, constructed from the thousands of classic herbal combinations. The most potent and traditional way to ingest herbs is to cook a raw herbal formula much like you would a soup. Another popular format is herbal powder, which you would cook like a tea, by dissolving the powdered herbs in hot water. Both the raw and powdered herbs allow the practitioner to customize a treatment for each patient. There are also pre-formulated herbal pills and capsules that are made to address common arthritis types. While these lack the advantage of customization, their portability and ease of use make them popular with patients. A good practitioner will be able to personalize your treatment by using several different pre-formulated remedies together. Additionally, since most herbs are imported into the country from China, you'll want to be assured that the herbs you receive are top quality and have been thoroughly tested for the presence of heavy metals, pesticides and bacteria.

First Line Therapy: Diet and Nutrition

Eating the right foods and taking the appropriate nutritional supplements are both extremely important in managing arthritis. With the right guidance, specific foods, proportions, and timing can be customized to fit anyone's needs. This type of attitude toward food also happens to be the foundation for a healthy lifestyle. It may not seem so at first, but making changes to your food choices and preparations can be easy and fun. It might seem like a lot of work if you're used to eating out or eating quickly, but most lifestyle changes are best done gradually and over time. Add one home-cooked meal here and subtract one food item there. Too many big changes can sometimes overwhelm you, so remember to make the changes at your own pace.

Within Chinese medicine, nutrition occupies a fundamental role. *The Yellow Emperor's Classic on Medicine,* a 5,000-year-old medical classic, proposed diet and nutrition as the first line of therapy against illness. Chinese medical nutrition focuses on understanding the healing properties of each food and pairing the food to the individual patient according to his or her therapeutic needs. Before a nutritional consultation, you'll be given a food journal to keep track of everything you eat and drink over a week-long period. This will help your practitioner to identify your problem areas and work with you to design a diet that incorporates the healthy things you already like to eat. You will also be asked to record your other habits and patterns, including how you exercise, your sleep cycle, and your daily energy levels. These can all help your practitioner to identify how your nutrition is affecting your life. In the case of arthritis, you will certainly be incorporating anti-inflammatory foods and avoiding inflammatory ones; those will only aggravate your condition. Be sure to work with someone who has received Chinese medical nutrition training and has been fully certified.

Visit Acupuncture.com for a list of Certified Chinese Medical Nutritionists.

Life Guidance with Wellness Coaching

Upon retiring from his long years of medical practice, Dr. Mao's father told him, "Disease is a symptom of life out of balance." Your sense of wellbeing stems from the health of each of the five aspects of your life—body, mind, spirit, finance, and relationships. When these areas are optimum and balanced you feel happy and well, but when any one of these areas becomes blocked or deprived, you will experience stress or trauma that can result in illness. Like many people, if this happens to you, you may choose to seek out a physician for your physical problems, a psychiatrist or psychotherapist for your mental and relationship problems, a financial advisor or accountant for your financial problems, and a priest or rabbi for your spiritual problems. However, none of the experts in each area can help you to integrate your life into a complete whole, which can lead to disjointed care. We recommend working with a Wellness Coach who can help you to discover your core self, find or affirm your life's purpose, and actualize your full potential by setting specific step-by-step goals and holding you accountable to reach each step along of the way. When you are living your life's mission you will feel happy and content, and your health will reflect those feelings.

Visit collegeoftao.com to find a certified Wellness Coach and begin your path of constructive life today.

Ward off Cold and Damp with Moxibustion

When the weather turns cold and damp, many people can feel it coming in their joints. For these types of arthritic conditions, ones that are worsened by cold and damp weather, there is good news. A treatment modality commonly used in Chinese medicine called moxibustion involves burning an herb called mugwort over a joint or body area to help warm the area and relieve pain. This heat-based therapy treats conditions where the energy or blood has become sluggish. Unlike a simple heating pad or other hot object, mugwort's medicinal properties allow it to penetrate deep into the body to stimulate blood flow, promote healing, and reduce pain. This procedure is usually done by a practitioner of acupuncture and Chinese medicine performing moxibustion with mugwort in a stick or adhered to the tops of acupuncture needles. For at-home self-healing, an alternative way to benefit from moxibustion is to spray mugwort extract on painful areas and apply a heating pad or infrared lamp to the area to help the herbal essence penetrate into the tissue for warming relief. See the Resources section for more information.

Bodywork Found to be Helpful for Arthritis

Studies have shown that types of bodywork, such as massage, have been shown to reduce pain from arthritis. In the Chinese medical system there is a comprehensive physiotherapy modality that includes a unique bodywork system called *Tuina*. Traditional Tuina bodywork combines massage, joint mobilization, and bone setting, and is often practiced by teachers of martial arts due to the frequent injuries suffered from their sparring activities. It works through the same meridians and acupoints accessed by acupuncture, and works specifically to unblock stagnant blood and relieve pain in the muscles, tendons, and joints. Tuina's history is rooted in solving the traumas associate with ancient daily life, including hunting, traveling, and building. Because the joint is a closed system, we need exercise and physical therapies like these to help push body fluids into the joint capsule. Toxins and other metabolic waste that make arthritis worse can be eliminated with Tuina. Be sure to ask your practitioner to incorporate Tuina into your arthritis-healing program.

Cupping Made Famous in America

In the summer of 2004, Gwyneth Paltrow arrived at the Golden Globe Awards with circular bruises on her upper back. This was a rather hip and famous time for cupping in America. Cupping, called *banki* in Eastern Europe, and whose use dates back to 3,000 B.C. in Egypt, can create bruises but there is no pain associated with the treatment. In fact, it's very relaxing and often a favorite of many of our patients. Bruising does not always result, and will only happen on areas of the skin where there is significant reduction in blood flow. The bruise is a release of old blood, allowing new blood vessel growth and blood flow to take precedence, and should fade after a few days. To perform cupping, a flame is quickly inserted into a glass cup, which burns up all the oxygen and creates a negative pressure like a vacuum. The flame is withdrawn and the cup is placed on the skin, creating suction and the feeling of a "reverse massage." Local tissues, blood, and body fluids are pulled to the surface. This relieves tension or adhesion in muscles and tendons, expels toxins through the skin, and stimulates localized healing. Cupping can be an excellent complement to any healing program, especially for the relief of arthritic pain.

Mind-Body Integration Through Movement and Meditation

Movement and meditation are important for health and healing and are essential parts of Chinese medicine. These may take the form of Qi Gong or Tai Chi, as well as sitting, standing, lying, and walking meditations. They bridge the mind and the body, unifying the two aspects of your being and accentuating your body's healing response. Determining which kind of movement and meditation are most therapeutic for your specific condition is best determined by your practitioner. Finding the right combination can align the body and the mind, setting both on a path to peace, healing, and wellness. Many studies have shown Tai Chi, Qi Gong, and other moving meditations can ease arthritis pain and stiffness. Joints are strengthened with the daily practice of these restorative exercises. While physical and mental stressors are commonly linked to disease, you can improve your health and rid yourself of pain and depression through proper use of mind and body. If your acupuncturist is not a certified instructor in Tai Chi or Qi Gong, go to chihealth.com for a list of certified instructors or check with your local YMCA or yoga studios for information on classes in your area.

Medical Qi Gong for Maximum Healing Potential

Qi Gong is translated as "energy work" and is a unique type of moving meditation that promotes mind-body integration for health, healing and inner peace. There are two ways to experience the power of Qi Gong; you can learn a Qi Gong form and practice it regularly, or you can receive treatment from a trained medical Qi Gong practitioner. Examples of self-paced practice Qi Gong forms include Self-Healing Qi Gong, Crane Style Qi Gong, and Eight Treasures Qi Gong. The InfiniChi energy healing system represents the latter type of medical Qi Gong treatments transmitted by the Ni family in the West. InfiniChi predates all other Chinese medical therapies and provides an energetic foundation to the practice of acupuncture, herbal therapy, and tuina. Medical Qi Gong gave rise to Reiki, another energy healing system. InfiniChi is a predominately non-touch healing system where the practitioner and the patient align their intentions toward a healing goal. In the case of arthritis, joint pain is reduced as the practitioner makes energetic adjustments, removing blockages and guiding the patient's energy to a pain-free balance point. The sensation from a medical Qi Gong treatment may be similar to the euphoria experienced after acupuncture, but unlike most acupuncture experiences, the practitioner stays in the room and spends the entire time working with your energy. InfiniChi is both subtle and powerful as it taps into and harnesses a patient's mind and body for maximum healing potential.

Choosing Your Acupuncture Professional Wisely

Most licensed acupuncturists are also trained in pain relief, as well as in the treatment of the diseases that frequently occur concurrently with arthritis, such as obesity, diabetes, cardiovascular disease, chronic illness and metabolic disorders. It should be reiterated that Chinese medicine as a comprehensive medical system is used as primary care for nearly two billion people in the world. An increasing number of people in the U.S. are turning to acupuncture and Chinese medicine because they're dissatisfied with their current state of care and are looking for a better way. What's more, many doctors are choosing to forgo setting up a family or general practice in favor of focusing on more specialized fields. When you start looking for an alternative to Western doctors, however, choose carefully. Only work with licensed acupuncturists (L.Ac.) who have graduated from accredited schools of acupuncture and Chinese medicine and are regulated by the state in which he or she practices.

Not all acupuncture practitioners are well versed in herbal and nutritional therapies, nor are they all proficient in tuina bodywork, medical Qi Gong, or wellness coaching. If a practitioner isn't competent in these other modalities, then he or she may be unaware of several potentially effectively treatment options for you. It is best to choose an acupuncture professional who you trust, with whom you have good rapport, and who has knowledge of a number of modalities. Some medical doctors also practice acupuncture under the name of *trigger point acupuncture, dry needling acupuncture* or simply *medical acupuncture,* which means they've taken abbreviated acupuncture courses, usually consisting of 300 hours or less, compared to the more than 3,000 hours of training required for a licensed acupuncturist graduating from an accredited university with a minimum of a Master's degree. This doesn't mean an M.D. cannot be a good practitioner of acupuncture and Chinese medicine, it just means that you need to interview practitioners before you can determine who is right for you. Go to Acupuncture.com to find a qualified acupuncturist in your area.

If You Must, Use Drugs Sparingly

Prescription drugs may have their place in joint care but relying on them as your primary source of relief comes with some significant risks. Drug medications for symptomatic relief of arthritic pain and inflammation include NSAIDs, or non-steroidal anti-inflammatory drugs, COX-2 inhibitors, immunosuppressants, and biologics. All of these drugs have side effects, including risk of abdominal pain, heartburn, constipation, diarrhea, gas, bloating, fatigue, headache, skin rash, ringing in the ears, anxiety, heart attacks, an inability to fight off infections, and toxicity to liver and kidneys.

The Federal Drug Administration (FDA) requires all drugs to be sold with a list of its side effects. This is a way of communicating the risks found during the drug's initial research and is helpful for physicians deciding which drug to prescribe, its recommended dose, and how to combine it with other drugs. But there is much that's kept from the public about the process of bringing a drug from the lab to your corner drugstore. The public is just barely beginning to hear stories of improper research methods, suppressed data, or entirely false claims, and unfortunately, in some cases, worsening diseases and even deaths after a drug passes FDA's scrutiny.

Nearly 200,000 Americans die each year from unintended side effects or complications from prescription drug use alone. This number is much higher than deaths due to street drug use or even automobile accidents. Much of the research that's done on drugs is performed outside the U.S. and all but completely absent of government regulation or public record. An independent news organization found 17,000 doctors since 2009 that have collected fees from pharmaceutical companies for prescribing specific drugs to their patients especially for off-label use. If you must use drugs, use them sparingly. Don't be afraid to question your doctor about its side effects, and don't stay on anything for longer than is absolutely necessary

Mechanistic Paradigm of Arthritis Care

When treating arthritis, conventional Western medicine uses drugs, injections, and surgery. All of these methods can include unwanted side effects and may prolong your rehabilitation time. Conventional medicine views the body like a machine. When a part breaks, simply replace it. While this mechanistic replacement model has many advantages, and can be necessary for those with chronic arthritis where the cartilage is worn or completely absent, for many arthritis sufferers the relief provided by surgery may be fleeting and result in more complications down the road. One recent study showed that knee surgery was no better than a placebo for arthritic pain relief. Conventional medicine alone isn't adequate to serve the 46 million arthritis sufferers in the U.S. alone, not to mention the hundreds of millions found worldwide. The key to lasting relief, prevention, and maintenance, is to turn to collaborative medicine and a team approach where both Eastern and Western medicine provide its patients with the best from each tradition.

Stimulate a Controlled Response with Prolotherapy

"Prolotherapy" is short for "proliferation therapy," in which a solution is injected in or around joints and connective tissue to aid in tissue healing and pain reduction. It's a relatively newer therapy, and only a few studies have so far been done to examine the it in full, but many patients swear by their regular injections for added relief. The solutions injected using prolotherapy are typically drug-free alternatives to the more commonplace cortisone injections. Things like sugar water, saline, animal cartilage, herbs, or homeopathic solutions are used to stimulate a controlled inflammatory response to help joints, tendons, and ligaments heal faster. However, pain relievers and other drugs are commonly used as well. Prolotherapy's focus is on the healing and inflammation-regulating effects of the chosen solution that is injected. Prolotherapy may not be appropriate for every arthritis patient, so make sure to discuss this with your primary care physician before seeking it out on your own.

Cortisone Injections and Oral Steroids

For several decades, the use of oral steroids or an injection of cortisone has offered quick relief to many patients with joint or body pain. However, the relief often wears off quickly and necessitates a prolonged use of steroids and repeated injections. What's more concerning is that many studies have found that some side effects from long-term oral steroid use include diabetes, osteoporosis and Cushing's syndrome, which is due to excessive levels of cortisol in the blood. Additionally, a recent study showed those who inject cortisone have an increased risk of a relapse of their original pain, and they tend to suffer from a markedly slower recovery rate, especially those who opt for multiple injections. But all is not lost if you've undergone this common treatment. Ask for a second opinion the next time you are offered a cortisone injection. You may want to seriously consider supplementing your arthritis treatment with the pain-relieving effects of acupuncture and Chinese medicine.

When You Might Need Surgery

While surgery shouldn't be your first choice, if all else fails don't foolishly suffer a degraded quality of life by not considering surgery if your condition warrants one. According to the American Academy of Orthopedic Surgeons, knee and hip replacements total 570,000 annually in the U.S. and this is estimated to increase drastically to 4 million by 2030. Surgeries for arthritis come with their own set of risks and complications, such as blood clots, tissue damage, and scar formation. This can put the arthritic joint in a similar state of pain and immobility as it was prior to the surgery. Additionally, the replaced joint isn't indestructible and it's possible they may wear down or break. All this could land the patient right back on the surgical table.

Both patient and doctor want to avoid treating the same thing twice. It should also be understood that a man-made joint is truly no replacement for the tissues you were born with. After a complete joint replacement procedure your ability to participate in heavier impact exercises like weight-bearing jumps or jogging will be extremely limited. Make sure to investigate all your options before getting a joint replaced. Sometimes surgery is unavoidable if the problem is beyond repair. In this case, utilize acupuncture and herbal medicine both before and after the procedure to prepare the joint and the rest of your body to heal and recover as quickly as possible.

Drugs and Herbs Can Exist Together

The science of pharmaceutical drugs really comes down to a single active ingredient. However, many of these patented active ingredients were first seen in nature. For example, aspirin originally came from white willow bark and coumadin came from turmeric. While science has done the work of proving certain active ingredients can work fast, the way the body uses and disposes of man-made products continues to be a problem. The body doesn't understand what to do with chemicals that have been stripped from their natural form, let alone chemicals that have been completely synthesized. Many studies show how drugs are taken into the body and expelled. But one would have to be studying the body's system in a holistic manner to know the number of reactions that cascade throughout when manufactured chemicals enter the body. We don't think a single study yet exists that manages to fully explain how the body digests, absorbs, and responds to a drug. Having said that, when drugs are used appropriately and in short durations they may offer relief to pain and inflammation.

After thousands of years of history and study, practitioners of Chinese medicine and acupuncture know which foods, herbs, and nutrients work well together and in what quantities. Many Chinese herbs contain hundreds of active ingredients working together synergistically. These Chinese herbs are almost exclusively used in combination with one another in classical herbal combinations and formulae, taking those active ingredients of a formula into the thousands. When battling a complex disease such as arthritis you need an army if you expect to win the war. These thousands of ingredients are often potent antioxidants which complement and assist one another, offering a comprehensive front when either attacking something in the body or nourishing and strengthening the entire body.

Doctors of Chinese medicine are trained in drug-herb and drug-supplement interactions. Consult your practitioner if you are taking pharmaceutical drug and herbs at the same time.

Putting Together Your Healing Team

While it is very possible to navigate your way through arthritis treatment with limited amounts of help, most people with chronic pain and movement issues will need to do one or both of the following: (1) Seek second or third opinions from people practicing the same medicine (2) Put together a team of complementary health professionals to assist you in forming a holistic education so your information is complete where it concerns both immediate relief and lasting wellness. When it comes to devising a team, we suggest that you start with a practitioner of acupuncture and Chinese medicine representing the Eastern medical paradigm and an internist or general practitioner representing the Western medical paradigm. The two specialists you will also want to have onboard are a rheumatologist and an orthopedist. A physical therapist can coach you in exercise and movement to help you avoid surgery, and can also help you to more fully enjoy physical activities, build better posture, or rehabilitate after a surgery.

Other important additions to your team include a certified Chinese medical nutritionist, a wellness coach, and a personal trainer well versed in Tai Chi, Qi Gong, and yoga. These practitioners will provide you with a customized eating plan to reduce inflammation and promote healing. They will help to identify blockages that may be causing frustration and an inability to move forward in your life, as well as training you in exercises that are suitable for your needs, to help strengthen you and increase your mobility. Once you have assembled the team that offers you the most comprehensive plan, it will be up to you to ensure that everyone is on the same page. Hopefully either your acupuncturist or your internist will also be willing to coordinate with the other members of your healing team, regarding the overall and specific treatment strategies and how members of your healing team can best work collaboratively.

Important Questions About Treatment, Drugs, and Surgery

The only way to find the answers you need is to ask the right questions. It is important to gather sufficient information in order for you to make an informed decision about your disease and find the treatments that are right for you. If you are unsure about the treatment you receive, try to have someone accompany you to your doctors' visits to be your advocate.

These are some of the questions you might consider asking: What are my treatment options? What are the side effects? How long until I see improvement? Can I expect a full recovery? What is my chance of relapse? How should I eat to speed my healing? What supplements are best for me? Is my weight optimal? What exercise is best for me? Where can I go for classes? Are there movements I should avoid? Does my job, living environment, or my hobbies need adjustment? Where can I get support for depression or anxiety? Will prescription drugs interact with my other medications? How long do I need to take them? What are the drugs' side effects? What can I expect once I stop taking them? How do I cleanse the drugs from my system after I'm done using them? Is there more than one drug option for my condition? Is there a natural alternative to taking a drug? Can I postpone the procedure? How long will rehabilitation take? Will I need other surgeries after? What's the chance of needing to repeat the procedure? Will I need drugs specific to the surgery or recovery period? Will I be pain-free? Will the surgery create more arthritis down the road? Can I expect to run, jump and be physically normal afterward?

The Future: Regenerative Medicine and the Need for Prevention

There is continuous research underway to build better artificial joints, stem-cell therapy to grow new cartilage, and ever-fancier drugs to reduce inflammation and stop degeneration. All of these solutions focus on making improvements to current available treatments for arthritis, and increasing quality of life for arthritis sufferers. However, with soaring medical care costs and the government's efforts to curb it, it is possible that we may not be able to afford the medical advancements after all, and will still need to look at alternative and more cost-effective ways of healing our diseases. In addition, more emphasis must be placed on prevention. It is important to teach both children and adults about how to properly care for their bodies and maintain their health. In the specific case of preventing arthritis, imagine if athletes were taught to use their bodies correctly; if they knew the biomechanics of movement for injury prevention, were taught the importance of healthy eating and nutrition to ensure strong bones and joints, and went through mandatory health screenings and check-ups to catch inflammatory processes at their onset, so they could be stopped early and therefore prevent the development of more serious ailments. Imagine too that practitioners of Eastern and Western medicine collaborated on treating patients as whole people and not just their diseases, taking into account their physical, emotional, and spiritual wellbeing while integrating treatment modalities that go from the non-invasive to the invasive as the need arises, all while emphasizing quality of life so that patients have the opportunity to achieve their full health and longevity potential.

Appendix

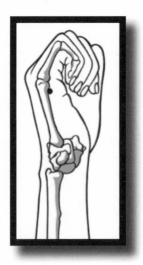

Diet Journal

	Sunday	Monday	Tuesday	Wednesday	Thursday	Friday	Saturday
Wake time:							
Breakfast Time:							
Snack Time:							
Lunch Time:							
Snack Time:							
Dinner Time:							
Exercise Duration:							
Energy Level (1-10):							
Bedtime:							

The Tao of Wellness Detox Diet

This is a cleansing menu that will work to rid your body of excess fat cells and toxins, allowing your metabolism to work optimally. This diet will normalize your inflammatory processes in order to reduce what's seen in Chinese medicine as Heat Bi arthritic symptoms, including red, painful, swollen joints. For those with mild to moderate RA symptoms, this food plan should be followed closely for no less than four weeks. For severe, chronic RA this type of menu should be followed indefinitely and will need to be incorporated into a comprehensive plan to overhaul your entire body. This diet is also very useful for Damp Bi arthritis.

<u>Upon Rising</u>
- Take 2 capsules of acidophilus or probiotic supplement. This will help repopulate the intestines with beneficial bacteria normally present in our system. These bacteria serve as a crucial part of immune function, but can sometimes be flushed out (along with any bad bacteria, fungus, virus, or mucus) when undergoing a cleansing, restorative eating plan such as this one.
- Drink 1 lemon squeezed into 12 oz. warm water. This stimulates your liver and bowel and is ideal before you begin eating for the day.

<u>Breakfast</u>
- A hot whole grain cereal (brown rice, oat bran or *Dr. Mao's Beautiful Herbal Cereal,* found in this Appendix) with 1 cup unsweetened, almond, soy or rice milk and a handful of berries. Start breakfast within 2 hours of rising.
- 1 cup *Internal Cleanse Tea*

<u>Mid-morning snack</u>
- 12 oz. vegetable juice and 12 oz. vegetable broth. The juice acts as a food-based multivitamin, providing you with all the vitamins and minerals you'll need. The broth is rich in chlorophyll and serves to flush the liver, kidneys, and blood of toxins, allowing in-

flammatory processes in the body to cease. Read on for suggested recipes for both the juice and broth.

* 1 apple

Lunch
Choose from one of the following options*:
* 1 cup cooked brown rice with steamed asparagus or broccoli
* 1 cup cooked brown rice with water sautéed shredded cabbage and bean sprouts
* 1 cup cooked brown rice with water sautéed bok choy and carrots
* 4 oz organic skinless chicken breast (Can substitute with turkey or tofu) with kale and mushrooms
* 1 cup cooked brown rice, ½ cup cooked black beans with steamed zucchini or cauliflower and 4 oz firm tofu steak
* 1 baked yam or sweet potato with sautéed chard (or any green leafy vegetable like kale, spinach, or collard greens)

*You may add to the above options: pinch of salt or pepper, 1 tablespoon of walnut oil, cilantro, parsley, basil, rosemary, oregano, lemongrass, or dulse (seaweed) flakes.

And: 1 cup *Internal Cleanse tea*

Afternoon snack
* 12 oz. vegetable juice and 12 oz. vegetable broth
* 1 apple

Dinner
* Choose from one of the lunch options. Preferably, you should have your evening meal no less than 3 hours prior to bedtime.
* 1 cup *Internal Cleanse tea*

Avoid: Alcohol, caffeine, wheat, refined sugar, deep fried, greasy, and fatty foods, dairy, nightshade vegetables (potatoes, tomatoes, eggplant, and bell peppers), spicy foods, and shell fish.

Detox Broth: Add as many of these ingredients as you can find at your local farmer's market or organic grocer into a large pot of filtered water: collards, Swiss chard, kale, mustard greens, cabbage, dandelion, Brussels sprouts, daikon radish, watercress, seaweed, shiitake mushrooms, cilantro, garlic, leeks, fresh fennel, anise, and turmeric. Bring to a boil and then simmer for an hour or two. You can make this broth in a large batch and refrigerate for up to a week.

Detox Juice: You can buy this from a store or juice bar, or you can make it yourself at home with a juicer. Remember to buy organic, and wash the following ingredients before juicing: carrot (with greens), cabbage, celery, cucumber, parsley, spinach, kale, beet and greens, apple, lemon, and ginger. Add 2 oz organic aloe juice to the detox juice. It's best to make it daily for maximum freshness.

Yeast-Free Diet

Foods to Eat

Vegetables: Broccoli, cauliflower, Brussels sprouts, cabbage, spinach, collards, chard, kale, mustard greens, parsley, dandelion, arugula and other salad greens, zucchini, squash, pumpkins, celery, asparagus, turnip, string beans, sweet potato/yam, radish, cucumber, artichoke, bok choy

Beans and Legumes: Soy beans, black beans, kidney beans, lima beans, pinto beans, azuki beans, mung beans, lentils, split pea, chick peas, navy beans, cooked peanuts

Dairy and Eggs: Eggs, goat milk, goat cheese, goat yogurt

Whole Grains: Brown rice, quinoa, amaranth, millet, barley, couscous, buckwheat, oatmeal, and corn

Unprocessed Seeds and Nuts: Almonds, pine nuts, chestnuts, walnuts, cashews, Brazil nuts, sunflower seeds, pumpkin seeds, flax seeds, sesame seeds

Oils: Olive oil, walnut oil, sesame oil, flax seed oil

Seaweed: Hijiki, kombu, nori, wakame, aramae

Herbs, Spices and Condiments: Ginger, cinnamon, pepper, horseradish, garlic, onion, clove, basil, coriander, dill, oregano, cilantro, thyme, rosemary, sage, bay leaf, mint, turmeric, cardamom, fennel, anise, green tea, stevia (for sweetening)

Foods to Avoid: Brewer's yeast, chocolate, coffee, all sweeteners (including sugar, honey, maple syrup, Equal, corn syrup, evaporated cane juice, Splenda and sucralose), alcohol, mushrooms, vinegar, dairy products (including milk, cheese, yogurt and ice cream, but excluding goat or sheep's dairy), yeast in any form, (including most breads and pasta), soy sauce and all fermented products like sauerkraut and pickles, processed meats that contain sodium nitrites, hydrogenated or partially hydrogenated oils, fruit in any form (including fresh, canned, dried, or frozen), and all processed and refined foods.

One-Day Fasting Protocol

- 1 lemon squeezed in 12 oz. warm water. Drink first thing after waking in the morning.
- Vegetable Juice: 24 oz. juice made from cabbage, cucumber, carrot (with greens), celery, turnip, asparagus, beet and greens, parsley, apple, aloe vera, ginger root. (Split up into 3 portions and drink throughout the day.)
- Vegetable Broth: 24 oz. broth made from as many of the following items as possible: collards, swiss chard, kale, mustard greens, cabbage, dandelion, Brussels sprouts, daikon radish, watercress, seaweed (any type), shiitake mushroom, cilantro, garlic, leek, fennel (¼ teaspoon), anise (1-2 pieces), ginger (3 slices), turmeric (¼ teaspoon). Divide into 3 portions and consume throughout the day.
- 3 cups of herbal tea throughout the day (*Internal Cleanse Tea* recommended. See the Resources section.)
- Supplement with 1 tablespoon of either flax seed oil or deep sea fish oil.
- 1 cup of liquid before bed time: 8 oz warm water with 1 teaspoon baking soda

Dr. Mao's Beautiful Hot Herbal Cereal

A nourishing and satisfying hot cereal made with herbs, grains, and seeds for sustained life-force energy (chi). Dr. Mao's cereal includes select Chinese herbs to promote long life; grains, legumes and beans for healthy digestion; and herbs and seeds for beautiful hair and skin.

Naturally gluten-free ingredients: Use equal portions of each ingredient: whole grain brown rice, mung beans, dried chestnuts, long-grain white rice, white lotus seeds, black rice, oats, green lentils, red lentils, black beans, millet, black sesame seeds, dried fox nuts, small red beans, red kidney beans, white beans, green split peas, black-eyed peas, yellow split peas, lima beans, pink beans, pinto beans, poria cocos, wild yam root, and goji berries.

Easy Preparation: Bring six cups of water to a boil. Add 1 cup of dry cereal mixture and simmer gently in a covered pot for at least two hours. You may choose to add agave, honey, or maple syrup for extra sweetness. Some prefer to make the cereal as a savory mixture by adding chili spices and seasoning. This recipe can be doubled or tripled.

Spice up Your Moves: Herb and Spice Blend

Mix together equal parts of the following: dried basil, cracked black pepper, ground cinnamon, chili powder, cloves, curry, fennel, marjoram, nutmeg, oregano, rosemary, sage, tarragon, and thyme.

Sample Arthritis Diet

The following nutritional guidelines are presented to show you how to eat your way to better health and pain relief. You may find that it's easier than you thought to follow these plans, a week at a time, and gradually build beyond that while continuing to emphasize the foods on these lists.

Appropriate food selection can help to slow the degeneration of cartilage in osteoarthritis sufferers and can also play a big part in helping rebuild cartilage to quell discomfort and improve joint movement. Anti-inflammatory foods make up a large part of this list as well.

Choose 3 meals and 2-3 snacks from the lists below.

Breakfast, Lunch, or Dinner
   • Two hard- or soft-boiled eggs. Toast from millet or brown rice bread topped with almond butter.
   • Scrambled eggs with spinach and chopped leeks.
   • Dr. Mao's Beautiful Hot Herbal Cereal, or a combination of millet and quinoa with unsweetened plain soy/rice milk, berries, and walnuts or sunflower seeds.
   • One or two turkey sausages. Sliced cucumbers with dash of thyme or rosemary
   • Broil Brussels sprouts, broccoli, and cauliflower by cutting in half, brushing with olive oil, topping with a dash of salt and pepper and broiling uncovered for 10-15 minutes. Serve with mashed sweet potatoes and spinach sautéed in crushed garlic and water.
   • 1 cup Salmon salad, mixing low-sodium canned or freshly cooked salmon, mayonnaise, chopped green beans, garlic powder, salt, pepper, and oregano. Serve with steamed chard and mushrooms.
   • In a slow cooker overnight, mix 1 part brown rice, 6 parts water, one piece of ginger, ½ chopped onion and a couple pieces of ox tail (ask your butcher for it) for a joint-healing stew. Garnish with parsley. Serve with collard greens splashed with apple cider vinegar.
   • Cabbage salad: mix together 1 tablespoon rice vinegar, 1 ta-

blespoon walnut oil, 1 tablespoon creamy peanut butter, 1 teaspoon soy sauce, 1 teaspoon minced ginger root, and 1 teaspoon crushed garlic. Toss that over 1 ½ cups sliced green cabbage and ½ cup sliced red cabbage, ½ sliced pepper (red, orange, green or yellow), 1 julienned carrot, 1 chopped green onion, and ¼ cup chopped cilantro. Serve with steamed chicken breast or shred the chicken and mix into salad.

Mid-morning and mid-afternoon snacks
- 1 cup goat yogurt with pumpkin seeds and chopped grapes
- Split one avocado and remove the pit, filling the center with balsamic vinegrette, walnut oil, salt, and pepper. Eat with a spoon.
- One apple, papaya, or bowl of cherries
- Sardines on brown rice crackers
- Black beans with cilantro and cayenne pepper
- One yam sprinkled with cinnamon

Additional Choices
Spices & Herbs: turmeric, basil, mint, cloves, green tea
Fruit: pineapple, kiwi, guava, kumquat, pomegranate, black currants
Vegetables: fennel, rhubarb, pumpkin
Nuts, Seeds & Beans: hazelnuts, flax seeds, soy beans, mung beans, lentils, split peas, kidney beans
Oils: olive oil, rice brain oil, grape seed oil
Fish: cod, halibut, herring, striped bass, snapper

Painful Obstruction (Bi Arthritis) Diets

Wind Bi Diet

Anxiety, excitement, and other unchecked emotions can stagnate your energy to the point where your nerves no longer fire properly. This can leave your joints open to the influence of weather outside the body and to the malfunctioning immune system inside the body. Physical rest, mental calm, and nutritional focus are the foundations on which you can rebuild your joints when Wind Bi manifests pain that comes and goes or moves around quickly, just like the wind in the trees.

Barley Ginger Cereal: Soak 1 cup of pearl barley overnight. Cook pearl barley with 9 grams of dried ginger in 3 cups of water over low flame for about 30 minutes. Remove from flame and sweeten with 2 tablespoons of barley malt.

Roasted Yam and Kale Salad: Preheat oven to 400 degrees. Dice 2 yams into one-inch cubes. Toss yam cubes in a bowl with 2 tablespoons of olive oil and a sprinkling of salt and pepper. Arrange evenly on a baking sheet and bake until yams are tender, about 20-25 minutes. Cool in the refrigerator until room temperature. In a second pan, stir fry 1 tablespoon olive oil, 1 sliced onion, and 3 cloves of minced garlic over medium heat until the onion is caramelized, approximately 5-10 minutes. Tear 1 bunch of kale into bite-sized pieces and add to the stir fry, cooking until the leaves are tender, approximately another 5 minutes. Transfer into a separate bowl and allow to cool to room temperature in the fridge. Once both the kale and potatoes are cooled, combine both mixtures in a bowl with 2 tablespoons red wine vinegar, 1 teaspoon chopped fresh or dried thyme. Add more salt and pepper to taste and stir gently.

Quinoa & Black Beans: Soak ½ cup black beans overnight. Drain and rinse beans. Cover beans with water in a pan. Bring to a boil. Reduce heat to simmer and cook until beans are tender, about 1-2 hours. Drain and put beans aside. In another saucepan, stir fry 1 teaspoon rice bran oil with ½ chopped onion and 1-2 garlic cloves until onions are light brown. Add ½ cup quinoa and 1 cup vegetable or chicken broth, or water. Add salt and pepper to taste, ½ teaspoon ground cumin, and a dash or two of cayenne pepper. Stir once, cover with a lid, bring mixture to a boil, reduce heat and simmer for 20 minutes. Stir in ½ cup fresh or frozen corn kernels. Let simmer 5 more minutes. Remove from heat and mix in black beans and ¼ cup chopped cilantro.

Black Sesame Crusted Halibut: Season the halibut fillet with salt and pepper. Spread black sesame seeds on a plate. Lay down the halibut on the seeds, pressing down to coat the fish in the sesame seeds. Heat a pan over high heat until very hot. Thinly coat the bottom of the pan with rice bran oil. Lay the fillet on top, seeds side down. It should sizzle loudly. Sear the seeded side of the fish for 2-3 minutes. Flip the fish over once the meat starts to turn opaque white. Sear the other side 3-4 minutes. A thicker fillet may take longer to cook. You will know the fish is done when the inside is barely cooked through. Garnish with lemon juice, a drizzle of olive oil, and chopped parsley. Serve with asparagus and mango salsa.

Other Snacks and Sides: scallions, grapes, celery, basil, sage, fennel, anise, oat, pine nut, coconut, chamomile tea, parsley, alfalfa, collard greens, lettuce, seaweed, black sesame, chrysanthemum tea, flax seed, grapefruit, daikon radish, mustard greens, pumpkin, turnip, azuki bean, millet, cardamom, cinnamon, clove, dried papaya, and rice wine.

Damp Bi Diet

A customized nutrition plan can help bring relief to those with Damp Bi arthritis. A joint has its own micro-metabolism and the following foods will help to improve fluid circulation and remove congestion to alleviate your fixed, joint cramps. In time, you may notice the weather doesn't affect your joints as easily anymore.

Mushroom Barley Pilaf: In a large saucepan, heat 1 tablespoon rice bran oil. Sauté 2 chopped onions and 2 minced garlic cloves until the onions are browned, about 5-8 minutes. Add 2 cups (soaked overnight) of Job's Tears (Chinese pearl barley) or barley with the soaking water. Next, add 2 large sliced carrots, 4 sliced celery ribs, ½ cup loosely packed and rinsed dried mushrooms, and 2 bay leaves. Stir well, bring to a boil, and simmer in the covered pan until the barley is tender, about 45 minutes. Turn off the heat and let stand for 10 minutes. Fluff with fork. Remove bay leaves and add a pinch of salt to taste.

Squash Aduki Bean Corn Chowder: Soak 1 ½ cups aduki beans overnight. Drain and rinse the beans and set aside. In a large soup pot, pour 1 tablespoon rice bran oil over 2 medium-sized, pre-rinsed, sliced leeks (or 3 cups chopped onions) and stir fry for 2 minutes. Add 4 cups of vegetable stock or water, the aduki beans, and 2 teaspoons of dried tarragon or thyme. Also add 1 ½ pounds of peeled and seeded butternut squash, diced into 1 inch chunks. Bring to a boil, reduce heat and let simmer for 1-1 ½ hours, until the beans are tender. Stir in 2 cups organic corn kernels (fresh or frozen), ¼ cup thinly sliced green scallions, and sea salt or tamari soy sauce to taste. Simmer 5 more minutes. To thicken the soup, puree a cup of the beans and stir back into the pot.

Millet Quinoa Porridge: Add 2 cups water, ½ cup quinoa, and ½ cup millet to a pan. Stir once or twice. Bring to a boil, reduce heat and let simmer for 25 minutes. Remove from heat and fluff with spoon. Spoon into 2-3 serving bowls. Add splash of goat milk, a pinch of cardamom, pinch of salt, and 1 teaspoon of raw honey.

Baked Stuffed Papaya: Stir fry ½ pound beef, ½ chopped onion, and 1 crushed garlic clove until the beef begins to turn brown. Add 1 cup of chopped tomatoes and a dash of salt and pepper to taste. Bring to a boil, then reduce heat to a simmer. Cook until most of the liquid has evaporated. Cut 2 papayas in half, remove the seeds, and fill the papayas with the meat mixture. Put papayas in roasting pan. Pour water into the pan, covering the papayas half-way up. Roast uncovered for 30 minutes or until papayas are tender.

Other Snacks and Sides: mung beans, mustard greens, sweet rice wine, cornsilk tea, alfalfa sprouts, artichoke, chive, parsnip, pumpkin, winter squash, turnip, tarot root, amaranth, pumpkin seeds, almonds, sunflower seeds, and fish.

Cold Bi Diet

Certain foods have a wonderful ability to warm up the body and the joints. Make sure to eat food that's warming in nature if you want to get the most from your food while dealing with Cold Bi. Additionally, chewing your food well and avoiding distractions while eating will allow your body to get the most out of what you're giving to it. Use the following foods and recipes as a guide, and continue to include foods like this in your diet until your relief is well established.

Lamb noodles. Cook wheat-free spaghetti noodles in water and remove when done. Grind 2 small pieces of orange peel into a powder and mix into ½ pound of ground lamb. Stir fry this mixture in a pan with 2 tablespoons of rice bran oil, strips of scallion, and diced ginger. Add dashes of soy sauce and cooking wine about a minute before the meat is well done. Pour mixture over noodles and serve.

Ginger yam. Poke holes in one medium-sized yam or sweet potato. Stuff holes with grated ginger. Wrap in foil and bake in oven at 350 degrees for 45 minutes.

Cardamom Chicken. Broil 1 medium size chicken without skin or organs with 1 teaspoon of cardamom powder and ½ cup of red azuki beans (soaked overnight) in an oven or pressure cooker in about 4-5 cups of water for 45 minutes.

Pepper omelet. Beat 2 eggs in a bowl with ½ teaspoon of ground black pepper and a pinch of salt. Fry in a pan with 1 teaspoon of peanut oil until well done.

Other Snacks and Sides: garlic, pepper, black beans, sesame seeds, mustard greens, rice wine in small amounts (unless you have high blood pressure), spicy foods, grapes, parsnips, curry, cinnamon, cayenne, freshwater fish, green beans, kale, mustard greens, parsnip, coconut, plum, tangerine, pine nut, walnut.

Heat Bi Diet

Inflamed joints can result from an injury or from other Bi types, if they go untreated. Make sure to eat from the following list to turn down any accumulated heat in your joints. Continue eating like this until the joints become less red, swollen, and painful. Make sure not to overeat at meals as that could make things worse. Pace yourself when eating and when healing, and be sure to drink 6-8 glasses of filtered water every day.

Sprouted tofu sushi: Sautee ½ cup each chopped onions and carrots. Add approximately ½ cup crumbled sprouted tofu and 2 tablespoons soy sauce. Mix together and remove from flame. Spread mixture evenly over sheets of nori seaweed, about ¼ inch thick, leaving at least 1 inch on each end uncovered. Roll up the sheets and place in a steamer with the seam on the bottom. Steam for 15 minutes. Allow to cool before slicing into ½ inch pieces.

Mung bean noodle salad: Boil water and pour over a few ounces of mung bean noodles. Noodles will be soft in about 5 minutes. While the noodles boil, soak several red dulse seaweed leaves in room temperature water for 5 minutes. Drain the noodles and put in a bowl with 1 chopped, seeded cucumber, 2 chopped carrots, and 1 chopped scallion. Separately mix together ¼ cup Japanese rice vinegar, 2 tablespoons toasted sesame oil, and dash of salt. Add to that ½ tablespoon finely chopped ginger. Pour this mixture over the noodles and vegetables. Drain and chop the dulse. Add it to the noodles along with ¼ cup chopped cilantro and ½ cup roasted peanuts. Mix all together and serve.

Braised bamboo shoots & bok choy in oyster sauce: Combine ½ cup chicken broth and 3 tablespoons MSG-free oyster sauce in a bowl. Cover a heated wok or frying pan in 1 tablespoon almond or walnut oil. Add 1 crushed garlic clove and 2 slices crushed ginger to pan. Stir fry on high heat for 15 seconds. Add about 8 sliced shiitake mushrooms and stir fry for 1 minute. Add 1 ½ cups sliced bamboo shoots and stir fry for an additional minute. Add the sauce and stir together. Lower heat to medium and braise for 5 minutes. Add 3 sliced baby bok choy and stir fry for 2 minutes. Dissolve 1 teaspoon cornstarch in 2 teaspoons water. Add to the stir fry and mix until sauce thickens.

Bean pita pockets: Preheat oven to 400 degrees. In a bowl, combine 1 cup precooked kidney, soy, or navy beans with ¼ cup finely chopped onions, ½ cup chopped tomato, ¾ cup shredded cabbage, ½ cup sliced canned artichoke hearts, 2 sliced tofu hot dogs, ½ cup soy cheese, and 1 tablespoon of your preferred salad dressing (Italian is recommended). Cut 4 whole wheat pitas in half, filling them with the mixture until ⅔ full. Wrap 2 pita halves together in foil and bake for 15 minutes. Open and top all pitas with 1 diced cucumber and ¾ cup mung bean or alfalfa sprouts. Stuffed pitas should be eaten immediately. Leftover filling may be refrigerated in a covered bowl up to two days.

Other Snacks and Sides: asparagus, beet, broccoli, spinach, squash, carrots, jicama, celery, corn, zucchini, cucumber, snow peas, water chestnuts, apple, peach, blueberry, strawberry, orange, cantaloupe, honeydew, watermelon, grapefruit, pear, asian pear, dandelion greens, cabbage, winter melon, green tea, and pumpkin.

Energy & Blood Depletion Diet

When your life includes excessive work, drastic changes in weight, chronic fatigue, severe injury, or long-standing illness, your blood and body fluids can become depleted, making it hard to keep the joints strong and healthy. When working to leave a state of weakness behind you, it's important to eat regular meals and snacks, never going too long without eating, even when there is weight to lose. Starving yourself or skipping meals will only make things worse.

Soft boiled eggs: Boil 2 eggs by cooking in boiling water for 3 minutes. Carefully remove shells. Serve with ½ cup cooked quinoa and ½ cup water-sautéed shiitake mushrooms.

Ginger-Tamari Salmon: Sauté salmon steak in water, 1 tsp. grated ginger, and 1 tsp. tamari soy sauce. If the water covers the fish about halfway, it should cook through in 4-8 minutes. The fish is fully cooked when a knife can go through it without resistance. Remove fish from water and drizzle with toasted sesame oil. Serve with steamed asparagus and yellow squash. Sprinkle vegetables with a little salt and pepper.

Turkey meatballs: Mix ground turkey with finely chopped spinach, salt, pepper, and garlic powder. Roll meatballs with your hands so each is smaller than a golf ball. Sauté in ¼ cup of water for 3 minutes. Turn them over and cook 3 more minutes. If all the water and juices evaporate, just add another ¼ cup of water. Serve with brown rice pasta and a small amount of tomato sauce.

Butternut Squash soup: Peel 1 large butternut squash. Remove the seeds. Cut into cubes. Put in a pot and cover with water. Boil for 20-30 minutes. The squash is done when a fork goes through easily. Drain the water and put the squash in a blender with one peeled kiwi fruit. Blend until creamy. If you want it thinner, add ¾ cup of unsweetened soymilk to the blender. Pour soup into bowls and crumble nori seaweed on top. Serve with side of steamed organic soybeans in the pod.

Other Snacks and Sides: goat yogurt, baked sweet potato slices, green beans, pearl barley, navy beans, cashews, pecans, pumpkin seeds, black beans, strawberries, watermelon, adzuki beans, pineapple, chestnuts, papaya, mango, figs, cabbage, carrots, pears, chicken, mung beans, buckwheat, jujube dates, beets, lychee fruit, and kidney beans.

Additional Recipes

If you need more recipe ideas, please seek the guidance of a Certified Chinese Medical Nutritionist. You can also visit Acupuncture.com for a list of qualified acupuncturists, naturopaths, and other professionals who have studied the healing properties of many foods and can devise a customized eating plan for your particular type of arthritis.

Cumin-scented Black Bean Dip: In a food processor, blend beans, 3 tablespoons olive oil, ½ cup plain low-fat yogurt, ½ teaspoon ground cumin, and ¼ teaspoon granulated garlic until smooth. Season to taste with salt and pepper and serve with carrot sticks, cucumber slices, or pita chips. Serves 4 as an appetizer.

Chipotle Black Bean Soup: Sautee ½ small yellow onion (chopped) in 2 teaspoons olive oil over medium-low heat until soft. Add beans, 1 smashed garlic clove, 2 cups chicken or vegetable broth, ¼ to ½ teaspoon chipotle chili powder (to taste), and a handful of baby carrots. Simmer 10 minutes, or until carrots are soft, then puree. Season with salt and pepper. Makes 2 small servings.

Black Bean and Corn Tacos: Combine beans and ½ cup chunky corn salsa in a small saucepan. Bring to a simmer, then serve in warmed tortillas, over baby spinach, topped with chopped avocado and a pinch of shredded cheese. Serves 2.

Maple-baked Black Beans: In a small baking dish, stir beans (with liquid) together with 1 tablespoon unsalted butter (cut into 4 pieces) and 2 tablespoons real maple syrup. Bake for 1 hour at 350° F, stirring once halfway. Serve as a side dish, or on toast for breakfast. Serves 2.

Black Bean Salad With Quinoa, Squash and Lime: Simmer ¼ cup dried quinoa, 1 cup chopped butternut squash, and ½ cup plus 2 additional tablespoons of water (10 tablespoons total), together for 15 minutes, partially covered, until the squash is cooked through and water is absorbed. Stir in beans, ¼ cup crumbled goat cheese and 2 tablespoons chopped fresh cilantro. Season with salt and pepper, then drizzle with lime juice and olive oil. Serves 2.

Roasted Soy-Ginger Salmon and Broccoli: By itself, steamed broccoli can be rather boring. But spiked with a mixture of soy sauce, grated ginger, and sesame oil, and roasted in a hot oven, it's sensational. Add some salmon, and you've got a quick, healthy dinner, all baked in the same pan. Place a ¾ pound piece of salmon, about 1" to 1 ½" thick, cut into 2 roughly equal pieces (skin side down), and 2 cups of big broccoli florets into a small, heavy baking pan or pie dish, snuggling all the pieces close together but not quite touching. Whisk 2 tablespoons low-sodium soy sauce, 1 teaspoon sesame oil, and 1 teaspoon freshly grated ginger together and drizzle evenly over the broccoli and salmon. Bake in oven at 425° F for 10 to 15 minutes or until the broccoli is tinged with brown and small white beads of fat begin to appear on the surface of the fish. Serves 2.

Nutty Rice: Rinse 1 cup brown rice and ½ cup raw shaved almonds and sesame seeds, drain in colander or sieve, and place in large bowl and cover with water. Soak overnight. In the morning, throw out the soaking water. In a pot with a tight-fitting lid, combine rice, seeds, 2 cups of vegetable or chicken broth and salt. Cook over high heat until boiling, then reduce to low and simmer 45 to 50 minutes. Remove pot from heat and let sit 5 to 10 minutes, then fluff with wooden spoon. Serves 2-3.

Sesame-Crusted Tofu: Cut 1 pound firm tofu crosswise into 12 slices. Place tofu in large nonstick frying pan over medium heat, cooking for 5 minutes on each side until lightly browned. Transfer to plate to cool. In a bowl, whisk together ¼ cup soymilk, 2 egg whites, and ¼ teaspoon salt and pepper until blended. On a large plate, combine 3 teaspoons breadcrumbs, 1 teaspoon each of white and black sesame seeds, and another ¼ teaspoon salt and mix well. Dip tofu slices into soymilk mixture, then dredge in sesame seed mixture. In large nonstick frying pan, heat ½ teaspoon sesame oil over medium heat and cook tofu slices, turning once, for about 3 minutes. Transfer the tofu steaks to plates. Trim the ends from approximately 12 green onion stalks, cut in half crosswise, then in half again before sautéing in a pan for 3 to 4 minutes. Use as garnish. Serve immediately with low-sodium soy sauce. Serves 4.

Broiled Miso Cod: Heat ½ cup sake on low flame and dissolve 3 tablespoons low-sodium miso paste and stir until liquefied. Cut 1 pound black cod into 6 equal pieces and place in a shallow dish, large enough so that all of the pieces of cod can lay flat in the baking dish. Pour half of the cooled miso marinade into the dish, add cod, and then pour remaining marinade on top. Cover with plastic wrap and refrigerate for 24 - 48 hours. Turn the fish every so often so that they get an even coating. Preheat broiler on high. When hot, remove cod from marinade and place on a baking sheet on the bottom rack of oven. Broil until caramelized, about 10 minutes. Turn cod over and broil until fish flakes easily, about 3 minutes more. Serve it with a side of brown rice. Serves 2-4.

Resources

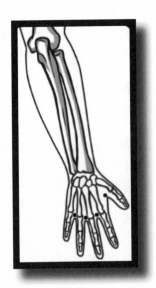

ORGANIZATIONS

The Tao of Wellness
Center for Acupuncture and Traditional Chinese Medicine
Santa Monica & Newport Beach, California
www.taoofwellness.com

The health center of Drs. Mao Shing Ni and Jason Moskovitz, the Tao Of Wellness is an integrated health, well-being, and longevity center that provides acupuncture and traditional Chinese medicine services. Each patient is viewed and treated as an individual whose well-being is affected by their lifestyle, diet, emotions, attitude, and environment. From the time you enter the Tao of Wellness to the time you leave, every staff member will be included as a part of your healing team. The center encourages the formation of a personalized, respectful, and trusting healing partnership. The Tao of Wellness' healing team highly values this partnership. The doctors are highly skilled in the art and science of healing, and believe in empowering each patient with knowledge and confidence. Their mission is to serve you, and to provide you with a complete healing experience.

The Wellness Living Store
www.wellnesslivingstore.com

This store is a valuable resource for a wide variety of healthy, healing, and life-enhancing products. It offers a collection of natural cosmetics; traditional Chinese herbal supplements; books on Eastern health and spirituality; instructional Tai Chi, Qi Gong and fitness books and DVDs; and meditation and music CDs. There are also lifestyle products including water filtration systems, a natural chemical-free cleaning system, and organic, chemical-free mattresses and bedding. Both avid learners and professionals alike will enjoy distance learning courses on traditional Chinese and western medicine topics, including some available for continuing education credits for licensed acupuncturists.

The Arthritis Foundation
www.arthritis.org

The Arthritis Foundation offers information and tools to help people live a better life with arthritis. Whether it's advice from medical experts to specialized arthritis self-management or exercise classes, the Arthritis Foundation has a wealth of information and resources to serve those suffering from arthritis.

Alternative Healing for Arthritis
www.arthritis-alternatives.com

This website is packed with information on well researched, evidence-based natural healing approaches to supporting patients living with arthritis. It includes studies on foods, herbs and nutriceuticals.

Chi Health Institute
www.chihealth.org

Tai Chi is considered to be the best exercise for arthritis patients, according to many studies. The Chi Health Institute is a non-profit institute that is dedicated to promoting health through the Taoist movement arts transmitted by the Ni family. Inspired by the teachings of the Integral Way by Hua-Ching Ni and his sons, Drs. Mao Shing and Daoshing Ni, the Institute offers professional level education and certification programs for Tai Chi, Qi Gong, and Taoist meditation. On the website, certified instructors are listed around the globe for personal coaching or movement classes. You can also view video clips of the exercises outlined in this book.

Acupuncture.com
www.acupuncture.com

An information-filled website containing everything you want to know about all the modalities of Chinese medicine, ranging from acupuncture, herbal and nutritional therapies to tuina body work, Qi Gong, Tai Chi, and meditation, complete with thorough research and a directory of licensed acupuncture practitioners throughout the U.S.

Yo San University of Traditional Chinese Medicine
www.yosan.edu

Founded by Drs. Mao Shing and Daoshing Ni in 1989, Yo San University is widely regarded as the premiere school for the study of acupuncture and Chinese medicine. It offers an accredited Master's degree program, and its doctorate degree program is in candidacy status. Yo San University provides low-cost and free acupuncture services through its community clinic, as well as in Children's Hospital Los Angeles, Venice Family clinics and Being Alive HIV clinic.

PRODUCTS

Water Filters
www.wellnesslivingstore.com

Filter out contaminates while keeping healthy minerals in the water. These highly-rated Aquasana water filters are available for the shower, the counter top, under the counter, and the whole house. Keep impurities out of your body and out of your joints.

Far Infrared Sauna
www.wellnesslivingstore.com

Great for most any joint pain, but especially Cold or Damp types of Bi syndrome. This healing wave of the light spectrum penetrates deep under the skin, breaking the chemical bonds between the cells of the body and those of harmful toxins and metabolic waste products, releasing toxins and chemicals out through your pores. The capability of an infrared sauna to rid the body of cholesterol, heavy metals, and chemicals is far superior to the sweat that's released from a typical hot sauna.

Arthritis/Joint formula
www.wellnesslivingstore.com

This Chinese herbal formula supports healthy joint function and the body's own pain-fighting functions. Used traditionally by Chinese athletes, people with joint problems, and the elderly, Arthritis/Joint contains eucommia, myrrh, and safflower.

DuraBone formula
www.wellnesslivingstore.com

A traditional Chinese herbal formula that supports your body's natural bone strengthening functions. Used by Chinese women for thousands of years, it includes Chinese herbs like Dong quai, eleuthero or Siberian ginseng, and astragalus root.

Pain formula
www.wellnesslivingstore.com

An herbal formula that supports healthy blood and qi circulation, as well as the body's natural pain-fighting functions. It also helps to expel wind, damp and cold Bi, and includes Chinese herbs such as peony, angelica, and frankincense.

Muscle Strength
www.wellnesslivingstore.com

This herbal formula is useful for building muscle and increasing stamina, including muscle weakness following stroke, myelopathy or sciatica. In Traditional Chinese Medicine, this classic herbal combination is formulated to move blood and help dispel blood stagnation from Qi and Yang deficiency.

Tonic Oil
www.wellnesslivingstore.com

An excellent general-purpose topical first-aid, this traditional formula activates the flow of qi and blood and provides temporary relief from aches and pains in the muscles and joints. It can also be used topically to support healthy gums, hair follicles and nails. Tonic oil contains oils of eucalyptus, fennel, and wintergreen, and makes an excellent bath oil.

Smokeless Moxa & Liquid Moxa
www.wellnesslivingstore.com

The herb mugwort is normally used in Traditional Chinese Medicine for muscle strains, menstrual cramps, and digestive discomfort in the

254 | Arthritis: Secrets of Natural Healing

form of Moxibustion (burning of mugwort sticks above acupuncture points, acupressure points, or areas of discomfort). As an alternative to burning the herb, and for easy home use, our Liquid Moxa tincture is sprayed on the affected area and warmed with a heat lamp, blow dryer, or heating pad.

Bone Health
www.wellnesslivingstore.com

Bone Health is a comprehensive bone formula designed to significantly increase the production of bone tissue. It contains a balanced range of nutrients including calcium, magnesium, vitamin D, boron, zinc, and other trace minerals.

Collagen Boost
www.wellnesslivingstore.com

Collagen Boost is a high-potency vitamin, mineral, glucosamine, and chondroitin formulation created to promote joint flexibility and mobility while strengthening skin, joints, ligaments, and tendons.

Super Vitamin A
www.wellnesslivingstore.com

Super Vitamin A provides a super concentrated daily dose of water-soluble Vitamin A in just four drops. A powerful antioxidant, it is used to maintain healthy vision, skin, and connective tissue.

Super Vitamin B
www.wellnesslivingstore.com

Super Vitamin B is a specialized and balanced high-potency vitamin formula with higher concentrations of the B vitamins that are especially important in combating stress and supporting healthy connective tissues.

Super Vitamin D3
www.wellnesslivingstore.com

Super Vitamin D3 provides a super concentrated daily dose of water -soluble Vitamin D3 in just one drop, and will support the absorption of calcium and boost breast, colon, prostate, and bone health.

Pro Omega
www.wellnesslivingstore.com

Pro Omega is a proprietary blend of polyunsaturated free, purified, whole-body fish oils that are extracted through cold press technology in order to preserve freshness and limit unpleasant taste. Contains Omega-3 fatty acids from fish oils, EPA (eicosapentaenic acid) and DHA (docosahesaenoic acid).

Eight Little Treasures DVD
www.wellnesslivingstore.com

This comprehensive 32-movement Qi Gong routine strengthens both body and mind. Grouped into eight "treasures" named for various aspects of our inner and outer nature, such as "The Great Bird Spreads Its Wings." Also included is a comprehensive foundation practice (or warm up sequence) that serves as a welcome regimen on its own. There are many exercises that lubricate and detoxify the joints through gentle, circular movements of the body. This well-rounded practice is easy to learn for participants of every level of experience or flexibility.

Meditation for Pain Management CD
www.wellnesslivingstore.com

Learn the mind-body techniques used by martial artists and Taoist monks that enabled them to endure and transcend excruciating pain. Throw pain away from your body as if throwing a ball. Abandon your limitations by outgrowing them. Overcome stiffness by mind-stretching your body as you've never been physically able to do. Use these simple visualization meditation exercises to aid you in the alleviation of pain. Draw on simple tools to keep yourself calm, peaceful, and focused. These are some of the simple techniques that you will learn from this instructional CD program for self-healing.

Meditations for Stress Release CD
www.wellnesslivingstore.com

Achieve a state of relaxation with these guided meditations narrated by Dr. Mao Shing Ni. These simple breathing exercises take no more than 15 minutes, but will help you activate your body's own healing mechanisms for greater immunity and prevention of stress-related conditions.

Tao Of Nutrition
www.wellnesslivingstore.com

Learn how to take control of your health with a good diet. The advantage in Chinese nutrition lies in its flexibility to adapt to every individual's needs for the prevention of disease and treatment of the whole person. Over 100 common foods, along with their energetic properties and therapeutic functions, are discussed, along with food therapies for many ailments, including arthritis, and many useful recipes incorporating these foods.

Tai Chi for a Healthy Body, Mind & Spirit
www.wellnesslivingstore.com

There are many styles of Tai Chi available today, but most of them focus on one aspect of its original purpose, usually the martial art or the health perspective, while the spiritual aspect is forgotten. This book presents Tai Chi as a powerful tool for cultivating the spirit, as well as the mind and body. This book introduces Tai Chi as it was originally envisioned and practiced thousands of years ago by the

Masters of Tao, as a tool for self-cultivation for the integration of mind, body, and spirit. Readers will also learn about the health benefits of increasing balance, strength and mobility with Tai Chi and be able to learn from the clear and concise photos and illustrations in the book.

Whole Food Liquid Vitamins
www.wellnesslivingstore.com

This highly bio-absorbable liquid whole food vitamin formula is made with organic ingredients and personally selected by Dr. Mao Shing Ni. A perfect vegetarian dietary supplement for you and your kids, just stir it into juice or your morning smoothie or drink on its own. A blend of veggies, fruit, vitamins, amino acids, antioxidants and minerals, containing organic noni juice and organic aloe vera.

Internal Cleanse
www.wellnesslivingstore.com

A traditional Chinese herbal formula that serves as excellent support for the Liver and Gall Bladder. Containing dandelion, peppermint, and chrysanthemum, the Internal Cleanse formula supports the liver's ability to cleanse your body of environmental pollutants, toxins, and excess medications. It balances your nervous system and relaxes your mind, and is available in tea or capsule form.

B-Slim
www.wellnesslivingstore.com

The herbs in B-Slim were carefully combined according to the principles of traditional Chinese medicine. It includes herbs such as sacred lotus leaf, hawthorn berry, and radish seed to reduce appetite and cravings, relieve bloating, support healthy digestion, a fast metabolism and balanced blood sugar, while gently encouraging bowel movement and elimination.